The *International* Classification of SLEEP DISORDERS

Pocket Version

Diagnostic & Coding Manual

Edited by the Nosology Committee of the
AMERICAN ACADEMY OF SLEEP MEDICINE

John Winkelman, MD (Chair)
Suresh Kotagal, MD
Eric Olson, MD
Thomas Scammel, MD
Carlos Schenck, MD
Arthur Spielman, PhD

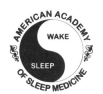

American Academy of Sleep Medicine · Westchester, IL

Recommended Citations

(Numerical)
    American Academy of Sleep Medicine. International
classification of sleep disorders, 2nd edition, pocket version:
Diagnostic and coding manual. Westchester, Illinois: American
Academy of Sleep Medicine, 2006.

(Alphabetical)
    American Academy of Sleep Medicine.
    ICSD-2 – International classification of sleep disorders, 2nd
edition, pocket version: Diagnostic and coding manual. American
Academy of Sleep Medicine, 2006.

Library of Congress Control Number: 2006922928

International classification of sleep disorders, 2nd edition, pocket
version: Diagnostic and coding manual. American Academy of
Sleep Medicine. Includes bibliographies and index.

        1. Sleep Disorders – Classification.
        2. Sleep Disorders – Diagnosis

ISBN: 0-9657220-3-1

PREFACE

This Pocket Version of the International Classification of Sleep Disorders, Second Edition contains the most clinically relevant sections of the ICSD-2, providing a guide for diagnosis of more than 60 sleep disorders. Diagnostic criteria are highlighted in a gray box at the beginning of each diagnosis. The essential and associated features, differential diagnosis, and subtype sections further aid in proper classification. ICD-9 codes issued in October, 2005, are also included. The version was edited by the Nosology Committee of the American Academy of Sleep Medicine, which included Suresh Kotagal, MD, Eric Olson, MD, Thomas Scammel, MD, Carlos Schenck, MD and Art Spielman, PhD. A comprehensive review of the final draft was provided by Michael Sateia, MD. We hope it will find a home in your pocket.

John Winkelman, MD
Chair, Nosology Committee

TABLE OF CONTENTS

III. Hypersomnias of Central Origin Not Due to a Circadian Rhythm Sleep Disorder, Sleep Related Breathing Disorder, or Other Cause of Disturbed Nocturnal Sleep

IV. Circadian Rhythm Sleep Disorders

V. Parasomnias

VI. Sleep Related Movement Disorders

VIII. Other Sleep Disorders

Pediatric Section

Abbreviations List for Pocket Manual

Abbreviation	Full Term
AHI	Apnea-Hypopnea Index
ALTE	Acute Life-Threatening Event
ASD	Acute Stress Disorder
BMI	Body Mass Index
CCHS	Congenital Central (Alveolar) Hypoventilation Syndrome
COPD	Chronic Obstructive Pulmonary Disease
CNS	Central Nervous System
CSA	(Primary) Central Sleep Apnea
CSF	Cerebrospinal Fluid
DLMO	Dim Light Melatonin Onset
EEG	Electroencephalogram
EMG	Electromyogram
GABA	Gamma-Aminobutyric Acid
HLA	Human Leukocyte Antigen
MRI	Magnetic Resonance Imaging
MSLT	Multiple Sleep Latency Test
MWT	Maintenance of Wakefulness Test
NOS	Not Otherwise Specified
NREM	Non-Rapid Eye Movement
OSA	Obstructive Sleep Apnea
$PaCO_2$	Carbon Dioxide Tension in Arterial Blood
PLM	Periodic Limb Movement
PLMD	Periodic Limb Movement Disorder
PLMS	Periodic Limb Movement in Sleep
PLMW	Periodic Limb Movement in Wakefulness
PTSD	Post-Traumatic Stress Disorder
RBD	REM Sleep Behavior Disorder
REM	Rapid Eye Movement
RERA	Respiratory Effort Related Arousals
RLS	Restless Legs Syndrome
RMD	Rhythmic Movement Disorder
SIDS	Sudden Infant Death Syndrome
SOREMP	Sleep-Onset Rapid Eye Movement Sleep Period
SpO_2	Oxygen Saturation by Pulse Oximetry
SRBD	Sleep Related Breathing Disorder
SRED	Sleep Related Eating Disorder
UARS	Upper Airway Resistance Syndrome

I. Insomnia

Insomnia is defined by a repeated difficulty with sleep initiation, duration, consolidation, or quality that occurs despite adequate time and opportunity for sleep and results in some form of daytime impairment. Among adults, reported difficulties initiating or maintaining sleep are typical. Concerns about nocturnal wakefulness or insufficient amounts of nocturnal sleep usually accompany these complaints. Less frequently, insomnia complaints are characterized by the perception of poor quality or "nonrestorative" sleep, even when the length and consolidation of the typical sleep period are perceived to be "normal" or adequate. Insomnia among children is often reported by caretakers and characterized by bedtime resistance, an inability to sleep independently, or both.

Insomnia is a symptom that often arises from primary medical illnesses, mental disorders and other sleep disorders. It may also arise from use, abuse, or exposure to certain substances. When the insomnia that occurs in these conditions is prominent, the reported sleep-wake disturbance warrants a separate diagnostic designation. Although selection of a single diagnosis is preferable, such a selection should not necessarily imply the absence of a subset of factors relevant to an alternate diagnosis. When criteria for multiple insomnia diagnoses are met, all relevant diagnoses should be assigned.

Standardized Criteria for Defining Insomnia
All insomnia disorders are defined by the following general criteria:

General Criteria for Insomnia:

A. A complaint of difficulty initiating sleep, difficulty maintaining sleep, or waking up too early, or sleep that is chronically nonrestorative or poor in quality. In children, the sleep difficulty is often reported by the caretaker and may consist of observed bedtime resistance or inability to sleep independently.

B. The above sleep difficulty occurs despite adequate opportunity and circumstances for sleep.

C. At least one of the following forms of daytime impairment related to the nighttime sleep difficulty is reported by the patient:

    i. Fatigue or malaise

    ii. Attention, concentration, or memory impairment

    iii. Social or vocational dysfunction or poor school performance

    iv. Mood disturbance or irritability

    v. Daytime sleepiness

    vi. Motivation, energy, or initiative reduction

    vii. Proneness for errors or accidents at work or while driving

    viii. Tension, headaches, or gastrointestinal symptoms in response to sleep loss

    ix. Concerns or worries about sleep

Diagnostic Criteria for

Adjustment Insomnia 307.41

A. The patient's symptoms meet the criteria for insomnia.

B. The sleep disturbance is temporally associated with an identifiable stressor that is psychological, psychosocial, interpersonal, environmental, or physical in nature.

C. The sleep disturbance is expected to resolve when the acute stressor resolves or when the individual adapts to the stressor.

D. The sleep disturbance lasts for less than three months.

E. The sleep disturbance is not better explained by another current sleep disorder, medical or neurological disorder, mental disorder, medication use, or substance use disorder.

Alternate Names

Acute insomnia, transient insomnia, short-term insomnia, stress-related insomnia, transient psychophysiological insomnia, adjustment disorder.

Essential Features

Adjustment insomnia is insomnia in association with an identifiable stressor. The sleep disturbance of adjustment insomnia has a relatively short duration, typically a few days to a few weeks. The sleep disturbance resolves, or is expected to resolve, when the specific stressor resolves, or when the individual adapts to the stressor. A variety of stressors may precipitate adjustment insomnia including changes or disputes in interpersonal relationships, occupational stress, personal losses, bereavement, diagnosis of a new medical condition, visiting or moving to a new location, or physical changes to the usual sleep environment. The resulting sleep disturbance may include prolonged sleep latency, increased number or duration of awakenings from sleep, short overall sleep duration, or poor quality sleep. Some individuals may present complaints of daytime sleepiness or fatigue, difficulty staying awake or repeated episodes of sleep during the day.

Associated Features

Sleep disturbance is the primary feature of adjustment insomnia, but it is commonly accompanied by waking symptoms as well. These may include anxiety, worry, ruminative thoughts, sadness or depression in relation to the specific stressor. Physical symptoms such as muscle tension, gastrointestinal upset, and headaches may also be seen. Daytime symptoms of fatigue, impaired concentration, and irritability may be attributed either to the stressor or to the sleep disturbance.

Differential Diagnosis

- Adjustment insomnia shares many symptoms with *psychophysiological insomnia*. It is distinguished from psychophysiological insomnia on the basis of its short duration, presence of an identifiable precipitant, and absence of a clinically significant learning or association component.
- Adjustment insomnia must also be distinguished from *circadian rhythm sleep disorders* and the *sleep disorders due to medical conditions* or *drug or substance use*. In each of these conditions, symptoms may begin acutely and may have relatively short durations. The distinction from adjustment insomnia rests primarily on the nature of the precipitating factor. In circadian rhythm sleep disorders with acute onset, the precipitating factor is an obvious change in the circadian sleep pattern as would result from jet lag or beginning shift work. Sleep disorders due to medical conditions or drug or substance use should be diagnosed when the clinician judges that the sleep disturbance is primarily related to that disorder or medication.
- Adjustment insomnia is distinguished from *mental disorders* by the severity of sleep disturbances relative to other symptoms. The acute onset, identifiable stressor, and short duration of adjustment insomnia distinguish it from most mental disorders.

Psychophysiological Insomnia 307.42

A. The patient's symptoms meet the criteria for insomnia.

B. The insomnia is present for at least one month.

C. The patient has evidence of conditioned sleep difficulty and/or heightened arousal in bed as indicated by one or more of the following:

    i. Excessive focus on and heightened anxiety about sleep

    ii. Difficulty falling asleep in bed at the desired bedtime or during planned naps, but no difficulty falling asleep during other monotonous activities when not intending to sleep

    iii. Ability to sleep better away from home than at home

    iv. Mental arousal in bed characterized either by intrusive thoughts or a perceived inability to volitionally cease sleep-preventing mental activity

    v. Heightened somatic tension in bed reflected by a perceived inability to relax the body sufficiently to allow the onset of sleep

D. The sleep disturbance is not better explained by another sleep disorder, medical or neurological disorder, mental disorder, medication use, or substance use disorder.

Alternate Names

Learned insomnia, conditioned insomnia, functionally autonomous insomnia, chronic insomnia, primary insomnia, chronic somatized tension, internal arousal without psychopathology.

Essential Features

Heightened arousal and learned sleep-preventing associations result in a complaint of insomnia and associated decreased functioning during wakefulness. The physiological arousal may be associated with emotional reactions that do not meet criteria for separate disorders. The arousal can also reflect a cognitive hypervigilance. Mental arousal in the form of a "racing mind" is characteristic. Learned associations are marked by overconcern with the inability to sleep. A cycle develops in which the more one strives to sleep, the more agitated one becomes, and the less able one is to fall asleep. Conditioned environmental cues causing insomnia develop from the continued association of sleeplessness with situations and behaviors that are related to sleep. Patients with this conditioned arousal may report that they sleep better away from their own bedroom and away from their usual routines.

Sleep-preventing associations may be learned during a bout of insomnia caused by other precipitating factors such as depression, pain, disturbed sleep environment or shift work.

Associated Features
The sleep difficulty often leads to deteriorated mood and motivation; decreased attention, vigilance, energy, and concentration; and increased fatigue and malaise. Despite these symptoms, individuals with psychophysiological insomnia do not show a tendency to sleep in the daytime, and many report an inability to take intentional daytime naps.

Polysomnographic & Other Objective Findings
Results of polysomnographic sleep monitoring may show increased sleep latency or increased wake time after sleep onset coupled with reduced sleep efficiency. Mean latencies on the MSLT typically fall in the 10-minute to 15-minute range, although a minority of these patients do evidence verifiable sleepiness

Differential Diagnosis
- Patients with *idiopathic insomnia* have an insidious onset of their sleep difficulties during childhood and endure a much more persistent pattern of poor sleep across their lifespan.
- Unlike *paradoxical insomnia*, psychophysiological insomnia is not associated with extreme and physiologically improbable sleep complaints or a marked mismatch between objective and subjective sleep measures.
- Psychophysiological insomnia has more obvious sleep-preventing associations and a longer duration than does *adjustment insomnia*.
- Psychophysiological insomnia should be assigned to those patients who show evidence of sleep-disruptive conditioned arousal as the sole or primary factor perpetuating their sleep difficulties.

A diagnosis of *inadequate sleep hygiene* should be assigned to patients who engage in activities that are inconsistent with good-quality sleep but show little or no evidence of conditioned arousal to the usual sleep setting.

- Psychophysiological insomnia that presents as a difficulty initiating sleep should be differentiated from *circadian rhythm sleep disorder, delayed sleep phase type*. In the latter condition, sleep onset is consistently later than desired because the individual's circadian rhythm is phase delayed relative to the desired sleep schedule. Also, sleep-onset difficulties persist, and sleep time is reduced whenever the individual chooses bedtimes and rising times that are too early and out of phase with the endogenous circadian rhythm. By comparison, those with psychophysiological insomnia typically feel tired or sleepy at the desired bedtime but are unable to sleep.

- Psychophysiological insomnia can be comorbid with other sleep and *medical disorders*. As such, psychophysiological insomnia may often be considered as a codiagnosis with another primary sleep disorder or with a diagnosis of other *insomnia due to medical condition*.

- The differential diagnosis between psychophysiological insomnia and *insomnia due to drug or substance* or *insomnia due to mental disorder* as the sole diagnosis is difficult, particularly when symptoms of anxiety or mood disturbance are apparent. Subsyndromal mood disturbance and anxiety are common in psychophysiological insomnia, but they are generally less pronounced than those seen in major mental disorders. Psychophysiological insomnia may be considered as a comorbid diagnosis when the insomnia precedes the onset of the substance abuse or psychiatric condition, follows a course that is independent from the associated substance abuse or psychiatric condition, or appears to be perpetuated in part by conditioning factors.

Paradoxical Insomnia 307.42

A. The patient's symptoms meet the criteria for insomnia.

B. The insomnia is present for at least one month.

C. One or more of the following criteria apply:

   i. The patient reports a chronic pattern of little or no sleep most nights with rare nights during which relatively normal amounts of sleep are obtained

   ii. Sleep-log data during one or more weeks of monitoring show an average sleep time well below published age-adjusted normative values, often with no sleep at all indicated for several nights per week; typically there is an absence of daytime naps following such nights

   iii. The patient shows a consistent marked mismatch between objective findings from polysomnography or actigraphy and subjective sleep estimates derived either from self-report or a sleep diary

D. At least one of the following is observed:

   i. The patient reports constant or near constant awareness of environmental stimuli throughout most nights

   ii. The patient reports a pattern of conscious thoughts or rumination throughout most nights while maintaining a recumbent posture

E. The daytime impairment reported is consistent with that reported by other insomnia subtypes, but it is much less severe than expected given the extreme level of sleep deprivation reported; there is no report of intrusive daytime sleep episodes, disorientation, or serious mishaps due to marked loss of alertness or vigilance, even following reportedly sleepless nights.

F. The sleep disturbance is not better explained by another sleep disorder, medical or neurological disorder, mental disorder, medication use, or substance use disorder.

Alternate Names

Sleep state misperception, subjective insomnia, pseudo-insomnia, subjective complaint of sleep initiation and maintenance difficulty without objective findings, insomnia without objective findings, sleep hypochondriasis, subjective sleep complaint.

Essential Features

The essential feature of paradoxical insomnia is a complaint of severe insomnia that occurs without evidence of objective sleep disturbance and without the level of daytime impairment commensurate with the degree of sleep deficits reported. The complaint of little or no sleep is accompanied by the report of extensive awareness of either the environment or mental processes consistent with wakefulness. The overestimation of sleep latency and underestimation of sleep time relative to values observed during concurrent objective sleep recording is a key feature of paradoxical insomnia. It is differentiated from other insomnia conditions by the magnitude of this discrepancy. In many cases the extreme degree of sleep loss reported appears physiologically improbable and inconsistent with the level of daytime functioning that such patients are able to maintain.

Associated Features

The patient does not exhibit features of significant psychopathology or malingering.

Polysomnographic & Other Objective Findings

Patients with paradoxical insomnia typically fail to show significant sleep deficits during polysomnographic recordings despite their reports of having slept little or not at all during these recordings. Standard sleep parameters such as total sleep time, sleep-onset latency, and wake time after sleep onset are similar for patients with paradoxical insomnia and individuals without sleep complaints. Sleep-stage distribution appears normal for most patients with this condition. Patients' estimates of onset latency and wake time after onset are at least 1.5 times the amounts shown by objective recording methods. Likewise, estimates of total sleep time are often 50% or less of the actual time shown by objective recordings.

Differential Diagnosis

- Unlike individuals with *psychophysiological insomnia*, those with paradoxical insomnia often do not show sleep-preventing associations that perpetuate the sleep disturbance.
- Paradoxical insomnia is not common in childhood and does not have the life-long course of *idiopathic insomnia*.

- *Mental disorders* can have significant associated sleep disruption that may contribute to the perception of little or no sleep. However, paradoxical insomnia does not share the other mood-related and vegetative symptoms common to these conditions.

Diagnostic Criteria for

Idiopathic Insomnia 307.42

A. The patient's symptoms meet the criteria for insomnia.
B. The course of the disorder is chronic, as indicated by each of the following:
   i. Onset during infancy or childhood
   ii. No identifiable precipitant or cause
   iii. Persistent course with no periods of sustained remission
C. The sleep disturbance is not better explained by another sleep disorder, medical or neurological disorder, mental disorder, medication use, or substance use disorder.

Alternate Names

Childhood-onset insomnia, life-long insomnia.

Essential Features

Patients with idiopathic insomnia typically complain of life-long sleep difficulty beginning in infancy or childhood. The specific nature may include difficulty falling asleep, repeated awakenings, or short overall sleep duration. The insomnia is persistent with few extended periods of sustained remission. One hallmark of idiopathic insomnia is the absence of any factors associated with the onset or persistence of the condition, including psychosocial stressors, other sleep and medical disorders, or medications. The baseline sleep problems of idiopathic insomnia may be exacerbated by factors that typically lead to sleep disruption or by the effects of medical or psychiatric conditions and medications.

Associated Features

Sleep disturbance is the primary feature of idiopathic insomnia. Psychological symptoms as determined by rating scales and inventories show only minor abnormalities in most patients with idiopathic insomnia. In attempting to cope with insomnia, the individual may develop behaviors that actually worsen the problem, such as excessive time spent in bed, preoccupation with sleep, or irregular sleep hours.

Familial Patterns

Evidence suggests the existence of a general familial vulnerability to insomnia, but it is not specific to idiopathic insomnia. Twin studies suggest a higher concordance of sleep difficulties in monozygotic than in dizygotic twins, although the extent to which this applies specifically to idiopathic insomnia is not known.

Polysomnographic & Other Objective Findings

Polysomnography shows sleep-continuity impairments involving prolonged sleep-onset latency, increased time awake after sleep onset, and reduced total sleep time and sleep efficiency. The percentage of time spent in different sleep stages is also altered with increased stage 1 and stage 2 sleep and decreased stages 3 and 4 sleep. Patients with some forms of insomnia show elevated physiologic arousal and metabolic rate before and during sleep. There is no indication that any of those findings are specific to idiopathic insomnia.

Differential Diagnosis

- During the childhood years, idiopathic insomnia can be difficult to distinguish from *behavioral insomnia of childhood*, in part because the long-term course of the disorder is not yet established. Idiopathic insomnia has no identifiable precipitating or perpetuating factors.
- Among adults, idiopathic insomnia must often be distinguished from *psychophysiological insomnia* and *paradoxical insomnia*. Patients with psychophysiological insomnia have stronger evidence for learned sleep-preventing associations or situation-specific arousal in association with sleep contingencies. Moreover, psychophysiological insomnia typically begins during adulthood, is more likely to have a discrete onset, and is more likely to vary in severity over time. Although discrepancies between subjective sleep disturbances and polysomnographic findings (if available) are present in most forms of insomnia, such discrepancies are clearly out of proportion in paradoxical insomnia relative to those observed in idiopathic insomnia.
- *Insomnia due to medical condition* can also present with chronic insomnia. Some of these conditions may have childhood onset (e.g., cystic fibrosis, neurodevelopmental disorders).

- Differentiating between idiopathic insomnia and *insomnia due to mental disorder* may be more difficult. Chronic mental disorders such as depressive disorders or generalized anxiety disorder may have early-onset, chronic sleep complaints and an unremitting course. The presence of other prominent symptoms of these mental disorders helps to establish the proper diagnosis.
- Individuals with idiopathic insomnia should be distinguished from normal *short sleepers*. Unlike individuals with idiopathic insomnia, those with short sleep do not feel particularly distressed, nor do they identify daytime consequences to their sleep patterns.

Diagnostic Criteria for

Insomnia Due to Mental Disorder 327.02

A. The patient's symptoms meet the criteria for insomnia.

B. The insomnia is present for at least one month.

C. A mental disorder has been diagnosed according to standard criteria.

D. The insomnia is temporally associated with the mental disorder; however, in some cases, insomnia may appear a few days or weeks before the emergence of the underlying mental disorder.

E. The insomnia is more prominent than that typically associated with the mental disorder, as indicated by causing marked distress or constituting an independent focus of treatment.

F. The sleep disturbance is not better explained by another sleep disorder, medical or neurological disorder, medication use, or substance use disorder.

Alternate Names

Insomnia related to psychopathology, psychiatric insomnia, insomnia due to depression, insomnia due to anxiety disorder.

Essential Features

The insomnia is viewed as a symptom of the identified mental disorder and shares a course with this disorder. However, the insomnia constitutes a distinct complaint or focus of treatment. The insomnia typically begins coincident with the onset of the causative mental disorder and waxes and wanes in unison with the other symptoms of this condition over time.

Associated Features
Difficulty falling asleep is typical in patients with anxiety disorders and is especially characteristic of younger patients whose symptoms meet the criteria for this diagnosis. In depression and, more generally, in older patients, frequent awakenings during the night and early morning awakenings with difficulty returning to sleep are more typical. Inadequate sleep hygiene and a history of multiple medication treatments for insomnia are also associated features.

Differential Diagnosis
- A diagnosis of *psychophysiological insomnia* may be more appropriate when the insomnia is largely maintained by conditioned arousal or learned behaviors, whereas *inadequate sleep hygiene* may be more descriptive for those cases in which poor sleep hygiene is the most obvious perpetuating mechanism.
- Anxiety is a common symptom of psychophysiological insomnia and insomnia arising from an underlying *anxiety disorder*. In psychophysiological insomnia, anxiety symptoms are primarily manifest as concerns about the sleep difficulty. In contrast, patients with insomnia due to an anxiety disorder manifest more pervasive anxiety symptoms that are not solely related to the insomnia complaints.
- Similarly, in psychophysiological insomnia, there may be dysphoric mood, lack of appetite, and other symptoms that may suggest a *major depressive episode*. In mood disorders, signs of depression typically persist even when sleep shows some signs of improvement.
- Many patients with insomnia due to mental disorder may display sleep misperceptions similar to those displayed by patients with *paradoxical insomnia*. However, the latter condition occurs in the absence of an underlying causative mental disorder.

Diagnostic Criteria for

Inadequate Sleep Hygiene v69.4

A. The patient's symptoms meet the criteria for insomnia.

B. The insomnia is present for at least one month.

C. Inadequate sleep hygiene practices are evident as indicated by the presence of at least one of the following:

    i. Improper sleep scheduling consisting of frequent daytime napping, selecting highly variable bedtimes or rising times, or spending excessive amounts of time in bed

    ii. Routine use of products containing alcohol, nicotine, or caffeine, especially in the period preceding bedtime

    iii. Engagement in mentally stimulating, physically activating, or emotionally upsetting activities too close to bedtime

    iv. Frequent use of the bed for activities other than sleep (e.g., television watching, reading, studying, snacking, thinking, planning)

    v. Failure to maintain a comfortable sleeping environment

D. The sleep disturbance is not better explained by another sleep disorder, medical or neurological disorder, mental disorder, medication use, or substance use disorder.

Alternate Names

Poor sleep hygiene, sleep hygiene abuse, bad sleep habits, irregular sleep habits, excessive napping, sleep-incompatible behaviors.

Essential Features

The specific behaviors that make up this condition can be classified into two general categories: practices that produce increased arousal and practices that are inconsistent with the principles of sleep organization. Commonly used substances such as caffeine and nicotine may produce arousal. Alcohol may also interfere with sleep by producing awakenings during the sleep period. Stress, excitement, demanding mental activities, and excessive physical activities may also lead to arousal and disrupt sleep when occurring too close to bedtime. Sleep may become disrupted or variable when too much time is spent in bed, when there is large day-to-day variation in the sleep-wake schedule, and when naps are taken during the day.

Associated Features

Inadequate sleep hygiene may contribute to mood and motivational disturbance; reduced attention, vigilance, and concentration; and daytime fatigue or sleepiness. Preoccupation with sleep difficulty is also common. Many patients with inadequate sleep hygiene show little insight into the effect of these practices on their sleep.

Differential Diagnosis

- Unlike patients with *psychophysiological insomnia*, most patients with inadequate sleep hygiene do not report better sleep in novel sleep settings nor do they show a conditioned physiologic arousal in response to their usual sleeping environment.

- Since sleep-hygiene practices may vary over time, patients with inadequate sleep hygiene show a waxing and waning of their sleep difficulty and are less prone to the persistent unvarying sleep disruption shown by those with *idiopathic insomnia*. Furthermore, unlike idiopathic insomnia, inadequate sleep hygiene is typically not diagnosed in young children.

- Patients with inadequate sleep hygiene may show a tendency to underestimate their sleep times, but they do not show the gross underestimates of sleep shown by patients with *paradoxical insomnia.*

- Arousal due to environmental factors may result from excessive ambient temperature, nocturnal prodding by pets, and excessive light in the bedroom. When these factors are the primary cause of the insomnia, a diagnosis of *environmental sleep disorder* is appropriate.

- Patients with moderate to severe *SRBD* or *RLS* may have difficulty avoiding daytime napping or adhering to a standard sleep-wake schedule due to excessive and pervasive sleepiness.

- Unlike those of *circadian disorders*, the sleep complaints associated with inadequate sleep hygiene are not eradicated simply by altering the sleep schedule to fit the endogenous sleep-wake rhythm. Furthermore, those with circadian disorders show decided preferences for atypical sleep schedules.

- *Insomnia due to mental disorder* and *insomnia due to drug or substance* should be differentiated from inadequate sleep hygiene. Various forms of depression may produce marked sleep variability or lead individuals to spend excessive time in bed so as to retreat from day-to-day stressors. Patients with inadequate sleep hygiene, like those with substance-dependence problems, may misuse substances such as alcohol in a manner that interferes with normal sleep. Patients with certain painful medical conditions may have variable sleep and daytime napping patterns as a function of the waxing and waning of their pain.

Behavioral Insomnia of Childhood

Please see the Pediatric section of the Manual for this diagnosis.

Diagnostic Criteria for

Insomnia Due to Drug or Substance 292.85 (for Alcohol use 291.82)

A. The patient's symptoms meet the criteria for insomnia.

B. The insomnia is present for at least one month.

C. One of the following applies:

    i. There is current ongoing dependence on or abuse of a drug or substance known to have sleep-disruptive properties either during periods of use or intoxication or during periods of withdrawal

    ii. The patient has current ongoing use of or exposure to a medication, food, or toxin known to have sleep-disruptive properties in susceptible individuals

D. The insomnia is temporally associated with the substance exposure, use or abuse, or acute withdrawal.

E. The sleep disturbance is not better explained by another sleep disorder, medical or neurological disorder, or mental disorder.

Alternate Names

Substance-induced sleep disorder, alcohol-dependent sleep disorder, alcohol-dependency insomnia, stimulant-dependent sleep disorder, drug-induced sleep disorder, substance abuse, insomnia related to drug abuse, rebound insomnia, medication side effect, medication reaction, food-allergy insomnia, toxin-induced sleep disorder.

Essential Features

Suppression or disruption of sleep is caused by consumption of a prescription medication, recreational drug, caffeine, alcohol, or food item or by exposure to an environmental toxin. Sleep disturbance may occur during periods of use, exposure, or discontinuation of the substance. Sleep disruption may arise from substances that act as CNS stimulants or depressants. Stimulants that most commonly lead to sleep difficulties are caffeine, amphetamines, and cocaine. Caffeine may cause difficulty with sleep onset or maintenance if consumed during the latter portion of the waking period or in excessively high doses throughout the day. The use of amphetamines and cocaine typically cause insomnia during periods of intoxication and elevated sleepiness during periods of withdrawal. Insomnia may be a side effect of certain antidepressants, various antihypertensive agents, hypolipidemic medications, corticosteroids, anti-Parkinsonian drugs, theophylline, anorectic agents, and a subset of antiepileptic medications. Pseudoephedrine and other preparations commonly marketed as nasal decongestants also may lead to sleep disturbances. Stimulant medications prescribed to treat attention-deficit/hyperactivity disorder or discontinuation of sedating medications may cause insomnia. Alcohol is commonly used as a sleep aid. Individuals who use alcohol to induce sleep may experience a reduction in sleep-onset latency, but they are more prone to experience fragmented and restless sleep. With prolonged use as a sleep aid, alcohol loses efficacy due to the development of tolerance. Extended exposure to environmental toxins are unrecognized for extended periods despite the presence of insomnia and other symptoms of toxicity. Common food allergies may also lead to difficulties initiating or maintaining sleep, or both, in susceptible individuals.

Associated Features

Insomnia resulting from excessive caffeine use may be accompanied by anxiety, jitteriness, and elevated daytime sleepiness. Mental symptoms may be predominant in chronic amphetamine and cocaine abusers. Chronic use of sedative-hypnotic medications may lead to tolerance, dependence, and loss of efficacy for some individuals. Abrupt discontinuation of medication, especially medications with a short half-life, may be associated with rebound insomnia characterized by a sudden worsening of sleep. Long-term use of alcohol as a sleep aid can lead to tolerance, dependence, and anxiety upon withdrawal. Since alcohol suppresses REM sleep, those who use alcohol as a sleep aid for prolonged periods often experience REM rebound characterized by vivid and disturbing dreams upon withdrawal. Many forms of prescription medications that have CNS effects may have disruptive effects on daytime functioning independent of the sleep disturbance they cause. In the case of food-allergy insomnias, other allergy symptoms may be seen. In contrast, those who develop insomnia in response to toxin exposure may develop memory loss, changes in mental status, respiratory problems, or cardiac symptoms. In addition, gastrointestinal inflammation may occur and lead to nausea, vomiting, and diarrhea.

Polysomnographic & Other Objective Findings

Polysomnographic findings vary as a function of the substance involved. Stimulants increase sleep latency and arousals and decrease total sleep time. REM latency may be prolonged, and total REM time may be decreased. During stimulant withdrawal, sleep latency is reduced, total sleep time is increased, and REM rebound may be observed. Studies of individuals who have used benzodiazepines on a long-term basis show relatively low percentages of stages 1, 3, 4, and REM sleep. Decreases in stages 3 and 4 sleep along with REM-sleep fragmentation are associated with extended alcohol use.

Differential Diagnosis

- Insomnia due to drug or substance should also be differentiated from *inadequate sleep hygiene*. Whereas patients with the latter diagnosis may display the inappropriate use of a substance like caffeine or alcohol too close to bedtime, these patients do not show the patterns of excessive use or dependence.

- A diagnosis of *psychophysiological insomnia* may be more appropriate when the insomnia is primarily maintained by conditioned arousal or learned behaviors, or both, whereas inadequate sleep hygiene may be more descriptive for those cases in which poor sleep hygiene is the most obvious perpetuating mechanism.

Diagnostic Criteria for

Insomnia Due to Medical Condition 327.01

A. The patient's symptoms meet the criteria for insomnia.

B. The insomnia is present for at least one month.

C. The patient has a coexisting medical or physiological condition known to disrupt sleep.

D. Insomnia is clearly associated with the medical or physiologic condition. The insomnia began near the time of onset or with significant progression of the medical or physiologic condition and waxes and wanes with fluctuations in the severity of this condition.

E. The sleep disturbance is not better explained by another sleep disorder, mental disorder, medication use, or substance use disorder.

Alternate Names

Sleep disorder due to a general medical condition, medically based insomnia, organic insomnia, insomnia due to a known organic condition.

Essential Features

Complaints of nonrestorative sleep are often seen in patients with chronic diffuse pain syndromes. Certain pulmonary disorders also may give rise to insomnia complaints. Obstructive lung diseases may be characterized by difficulty initiating sleep, frequent awakenings associated with respiratory distress (e.g., shortness of breath or nocturnal cough), and feeling unrested upon awakening in the morning. Patients with sleep-related asthma commonly show nocturnal awakenings with dyspnea, wheezing, coughing, air hunger, or chest tightness associated with anxiety. Several neurological disorders may also cause insomnia complaints because they lead to fragmented sleep patterns, subjective sleep concerns, and a disruption of sleep-wake cycles. Sleep disturbance in association with menopause is common and may lead to insomnia complaints; affected women are bothered by repeated nocturnal awakenings, associated with "hot flashes" or "night sweats." Pregnancy may also cause sleep difficulty, particularly in the last trimester. Frequent nocturnal awakenings and a loss of slow-wave sleep are common.

Associated Features
Insomnia due to medical condition may be associated with excessive focus on sleep, anxiety about not sleeping well, and complaints of daytime dysfunction. Worries about the effects of the insomnia on the causative medical disorder or condition or on health in general are not uncommon.

Polysomnographic & Other Objective Findings
Most medical or physiologic conditions that cause insomnia produce a decrease in total sleep time, an increase in awakenings from sleep, and a decrease in slow-wave sleep.

Differential Diagnosis
- *Insomnia due to drug or substance* should be assigned when it is clear that the insomnia began soon after the medication was prescribed and remits or improves when the medication is withdrawn. In contrast, insomnia due to medical condition should be assigned when the insomnia waxes and wanes with the waxing and waning of the medical condition itself.
- Additional insomnia diagnoses such as *psychophysiological insomnia* or *inadequate sleep hygiene* may be appropriate primary or comorbid diagnoses.

Insomnia Not Due to Substance or Known Physiologic Condition, Unspecified (*Nonorganic Insomnia, NOS*) 780.52

This diagnosis is used for forms of insomnia that cannot be classified elsewhere but are suspected to be related to an underlying mental disorder, psychological factors, or sleep-disruptive practices. In some cases, this diagnosis may be assigned on a temporary basis when an insomnia diagnosis seems appropriate but further evaluation is required to determine the specific mental condition or psychological and behavioral factors responsible for the reported sleep difficulty. In other cases, this diagnosis may be assigned when psychological or behavioral factors appear to contribute to the insomnia but the patient's symptoms fail to meet criteria for one of the other insomnia diagnoses.

Physiologic (*Organic*) Insomnia, Unspecified 327.00

This diagnosis is used for forms of insomnia that cannot be classified elsewhere but are suspected to be related to an underlying medical disorder, physiological state, or substance use or exposure. In some cases, this diagnosis may be assigned on a temporary basis when an insomnia diagnosis seems appropriate but further evaluation is required to determine the specific medical condition or toxin exposure responsible for the reported sleep difficulty. This diagnosis may also be assigned when substance abuse or dependence-related insomnia is suspected but is yet to be confirmed. In other cases, this diagnosis may be assigned when an endogenous physiologic disorder or condition appears to contribute to the insomnia but the patient's symptoms fail to meet the criteria for one of the other insomnia diagnoses.

II. Sleep Related Breathing Disorders

The disorders in this subgroup are characterized by disordered respiration during sleep. Central sleep apnea syndromes include those in which respiratory effort is diminished or absent in an intermittent or cyclic fashion due to central nervous system or cardiac dysfunction. The obstructive sleep apnea syndromes include those in which there is an obstruction in the airway resulting in continued breathing effort but inadequate ventilation. Adult and pediatric patients are identified separately because the disorders have different methods of diagnosis and treatment.

The term *alveolar hypoventilation* represents a physiological outcome of one disorder or a combination of disorders leading to an elevation of $PaCO_2$ above 45 mm Hg. This elevation, termed *hypercapnia*, reflects an imbalance between metabolic production of carbon dioxide and elimination of carbon dioxide through exhaled gas. Clinically relevant disorders that are associated with alveolar hypoventilation primarily limit the physiological ability to excrete carbon dioxide.

In addition, the chronic disorder must be distinguished from acute alveolar hypoventilation. The literature has not specifically addressed this distinction. However, it is reasonable to define the condition as chronic when the $PaCO_2$ remains above 45 mm Hg and there have been no episodes of exacerbation of the underlying disorder for at least one month. This definition does not preclude a slow, progressively increasing $PaCO_2$ over time, paralleling the course of the underlying disease process.

Because alveolar hypoventilation is physiologically defined by a $PaCO_2$ greater than 45 mm Hg and measured by arterial blood sampling, a procedure historically performed in awake individuals, this condition was initially recognized in the context of wakefulness. However, this definition is confounded by physiologic rise in $PaCO_2$ of 4 to 6 mm Hg that occurs during sleep even in normal subjects. Although there is evidence that alveolar hypoventilation during sleep may precede hypoventilation during wakefulness, the level of arterial $PaCO_2$ that demarcates the transition from physiologic hypercapnia to pathologic hypoventilation is not well defined. In view of the ambiguity of the terms *acute* and *chronic* in this circumstance, it is best to employ the general term *sleep related alveolar hypoventilation*, recognizing that the degree of hypoventilation covered by this term exceeds the expected physiological hypercapnia and that hypoventilation may or may not be present during wakefulness as well, depending on the nature and severity of the underlying disorder.

This classification is subdivided according to the underlying pathophysiological processes that are associated with sleep related nonobstructive alveolar hypoventilation. In this context, the term *nonobstructive* indicates the absence of upper airway obstruction during sleep (e.g., OSA). *Sleep related nonobstructive alveolar hypoventilation* can occur in an idiopathic form in patients with normal mechanical properties of the lung but more commonly is secondary to medical conditions that alter the mechanical properties of the lungs, chest wall, or ventilatory muscles.

Diagnostic Criteria for

Primary Central Sleep Apnea 327.21

A. The patient reports at least one of the following:
      i. Excessive daytime sleepiness
      ii. Frequent arousals and awakenings during sleep or insomnia complaints
      iii. Awakening short of breath
B. Polysomnography shows five or more central apneas per hour of sleep.
C. The disorder is not better explained by another current sleep disorder, medical or neurological disorder, medication use, or substance use disorder.

Essential Features

Primary central sleep apnea (CSA) is of unknown etiology (idiopathic) and is characterized on the polysomnogram by recurrent cessation of respiration during sleep with the apnea having no associated ventilatory effort. This recurrent cessation and resumption of ventilation can lead to sleep fragmentation, yielding excessive daytime sleepiness, frequent nocturnal awakenings, or both. Patients with CSA tend to have low normal arterial $PaCO_2$ during wakefulness (less than 40 mm Hg).

Associated Features

Primary central sleep apnea may be associated with snoring, witnessed apnea, and awakening with shortness of breath.

Polysomnographic & Other Objective Findings

The polysomnogram of the patient with CSA demonstrates recurrent (more than five per hour) cessations in ventilatory effort and ventilation during the onset of NREM sleep or, less commonly, during stable NREM sleep. These apneas are 10 seconds or longer in duration and commonly lead to mild arterial oxygen desaturation. These events are less common during REM sleep.

Differential Diagnosis

- In *OSA*, polysomnography demonstrates respiratory effort during apneic events, whereas effort is absent during central apneic events.
- During *Cheyne Stokes breathing pattern*, there is a crescendo-decrescendo pattern of breathing, whereas central apneas are generally terminated abruptly with a large breath.
- In *sleep related hypoventilation/hypoxemic syndromes*, patients with waking hypercapnia ($PaCO_2$ greater than 45 mm Hg) due to a ventilatory control problem, obesity-hypoventilation syndrome, or neuromuscular disease can have central apneas during sleep. However, in these conditions, there is commonly substantial oxygen desaturation secondary to hypoventilation, and desaturation is worse during REM sleep. Reduced waking oxygen saturation may be present as well.
- Central apneas in the wake-sleep transition can occur in *normal* individuals. However, once stable sleep is achieved, these apneas should cease. Normal individuals should not have more than five such central apneas per hour of sleep.

Diagnostic Criteria for

Cheyne Stokes Breathing Pattern 786.04

A. Polysomnography shows at least 10 central apneas and hypopneas per hour of sleep in which the hypopnea has a crescendo-decrescendo pattern of tidal volume accompanied by frequent arousals from sleep and derangement of sleep structure.

Note: Although symptoms are not mandatory to make this diagnosis, patients often report excessive daytime sleepiness, frequent arousals and awakenings during sleep, insomnia complaints, or awakening short of breath.

B. The breathing disorder occurs in association with a serious medical illness, such as heart failure, stroke, or renal failure.

C. The disorder is not better explained by another current sleep disorder, medication use, or substance use disorder.

Alternate Names
Periodic breathing.

Essential Features
Cheyne Stokes breathing pattern is characterized by recurrent apneas, hypopneas, or both apneas and hypopneas alternating with prolonged hyperpneas during which tidal volume gradually waxes and wanes in a crescendo-decrescendo pattern. As in other forms of CSA, apneas and hypopneas are associated with absent or reduced ventilatory effort, respectively, due to diminished central respiratory drive.

Associated Features
Presenting features of Cheyne Stokes breathing pattern during sleep may include excessive daytime sleepiness, insomnia, or episodic nocturnal dyspnea. It is also a cause of paroxysmal nocturnal dyspnea. However, a substantial number of patients with this disorder do not complain of any of these symptoms, in which case it may be identified serendipitously at the bedside. Cheyne Stokes breathing pattern can also occur during wakefulness, at which time its clinical significance is not as clear as during sleep.

Predisposing & Precipitating Factors

The most important predisposing factors are the presence of congestive heart failure, stroke, and perhaps renal failure. Within the heart failure population, risk factors for Cheyne Stokes breathing pattern during sleep include male sex, age older than 60 years, the presence of atrial fibrillation, and hypocapnia (i.e., awake $PaCO_2$ of 38 mm Hg or less).

Polysomnographic & Other Objective Findings

Cheyne Stokes breathing pattern typically occurs at the transition from wakefulness to NREM sleep and during stages 1 and 2 of NREM sleep. It tends to dissipate in stages 3 and 4 and in REM sleep. Arousals may occur at the termination of apneas, but, in contrast to other forms of sleep apnea, they often occur a few breaths after the resumption of ventilation. Many apneas and hypopneas are not accompanied by arousals. Apneas and hypopneas are usually accompanied by modest oxyhemoglobin desaturation; SpO_2 seldom falls below 80% to 85%.

Differential Diagnosis

- *CSA* can usually be distinguished from Cheyne Stokes breathing pattern by the absence of a history of heart failure, stroke, or renal failure and by the absence of a crescendo-decrescendo pattern lasting longer than 45 seconds.
- *High-altitude periodic breathing* only occurs at high altitude and is not associated with heart failure, stroke, or renal failure.
- *Sleep related hypoventilation/hypoxemic syndromes* can be readily distinguished from Cheyne Stokes breathing pattern by the presence of hypercapnic respiratory failure with a $PaCO_2$ greater than 45 mm Hg. Additionally, oxygen desaturation in hypoventilation/hypoxemic syndromes is generally more pronounced, particularly during REM sleep.
- *OSA* is distinguished by the presence of respiratory efforts during apneas.
- A few central apneas or hypopneas at sleep onset or during REM sleep are *normal* in elderly subjects. These cease once sleep becomes stable.

Diagnostic Criteria for

High-Altitude Periodic Breathing 327.22

A. Recent ascent to altitude of at least 4,000 meters
B. Polysomnography demonstrates recurrent central apneas primarily during NREM sleep at a frequency greater than five per hour. The cycle length should be 12 to 34 seconds.

Note: *Because high-altitude periodic breathing is a normal adaptation to altitude, there are no specific criteria regarding the frequency of central apneas that should be considered normal or abnormal. Although no specific symptoms are required, recurrent awakening during the night and fatigue during the day may be present.*

Essential Features

High-altitude periodic breathing is characterized by cycling periods of apnea and hyperpnea with the apnea being associated with no ventilatory effort (a central apnea). This periodic breathing occurs on ascent to altitude, with virtually everyone demonstrating this respiratory pattern at elevations higher than 7,600 meters and some at altitude lower than 5,000 meters.

Associated Features

At altitude, individuals may complain of frequent awakenings, poor quality sleep, and a sense of suffocation. This will often improve with time at altitude if the elevation is not extreme.

Polysomnographic & Other Objective Findings

The apneas are generally 10 seconds or longer in duration. This breathing pattern occurs only during NREM sleep with more rhythmic respiration during REM sleep. The apneas and associated hyperpnea can lead to recurrent arousals from sleep, which often increase stages 1 and 2 sleep, while stages 3 and 4 sleep are reduced.

Differential Diagnosis

- The major distinguishing factor is recent ascent to high altitude.
- On polysomnogram, patients with *OSA* will demonstrate continued respiratory effort during apneas.
- Patients with *chronic mountain sickness* demonstrate relative hypoventilation at altitude (i.e., breathe less than is encountered in normal individuals at similar altitude) such that they are more hypoxic than normal individuals who have a greater ventilatory response to the same ambient hypoxia. During sleep, these individuals often demonstrate further oxygen desaturation but rarely have actual apneas or periodic breathing. In addition, chronic mountain sickness develops over long periods at altitude, whereas periodic breathing is most commonly encountered immediately after ascent.

Central Sleep Apnea Due to Medical Condition Not Cheyne Stokes 327.27

Central sleep apnea that is believed to be secondary to a medical condition and that does not exhibit a characteristic pattern of Cheyne Stokes respirations is classified here. The majority of these patients are probably individuals with brainstem lesions of vascular, neoplastic, degenerative, demyelinating, or traumatic origin. Other etiologies include cardiac and renal disorders.

Central Sleep Apnea Due to Drug or Substance 327.29

A. The patient has been taking a long-acting opioid regularly for at least two months.

B. Polysomnography shows a central apnea index of five or more or periodic breathing (10 or more central apneas and hypopneas per hour of sleep in which the hyperpnea has a crescendo-decrescendo pattern of tidal volume, accompanied by frequent arousals from sleep and derangement of sleep structure).

C. The disorder is not better explained by another current sleep disorder or medical or neurological disorder.

Essential Features
The most common offending drug is methadone; however, the condition has also been described in patients taking time-release morphine and hydrocodone.

Polysomnographic & Other Objective Findings
A variety of abnormalities have been described, including central apneas, Biot's breathing pattern, and periodic breathing. Obstructive breathing events may also be more common in patients using long-acting opioids, but there are no well-controlled studies to confirm this.

Differential Diagnosis
This condition is best distinguished by the patient's ongoing use of long-acting opioids. Other sleep related breathing disorders may be present and may complicate polysomnographic findings.

Primary Sleep Apnea of Infancy
(Formerly Primary Sleep Apnea of Newborn)
Please see the Pediatric section of the Manual for this diagnosis.

Diagnostic Criteria for

Obstructive Sleep Apnea, Adult 327.23

A, B, and D or C and D satisfy the criteria:

A. At least one of the following applies:

    i. The patient complains of unintentional sleep episodes during wakefulness, daytime sleepiness, unrefreshing sleep, fatigue, or insomnia

    ii. The patient wakes with breath holding, gasping, or choking

    iii. The bed partner reports loud snoring, breathing interruptions, or both during the patient's sleep

B. Polysomnographic recording shows the following:

    i. Five or more scoreable respiratory events (i.e., apneas, hypopneas, or RERAs) per hour of sleep

    ii. Evidence of respiratory effort during all or a portion of each respiratory event (In the case of a RERA, this is best seen with the use of esophageal manometry)

OR

C. Polysomnographic recording shows the following:

    i. Fifteen or more scoreable respiratory events (i.e., apneas, hypopneas, or RERAs) per hour of sleep

    ii. Evidence of respiratory effort during all or a portion of each respiratory event (In the case of a RERA, this is best seen with the use of esophageal manometry)

D. The disorder is not better explained by another current sleep disorder, medical or neurological disorder, medication use, or substance use disorder.

Essential Features

OSA is characterized by repetitive episodes of complete (apnea) or partial (hypopnea) upper airway obstruction occurring during sleep. These events often result in reductions in blood oxygen saturation and are usually terminated by brief arousals from sleep. By definition, apneic and hypopneic events last a minimum of 10 seconds. Events can occur in any stage of sleep but more frequently occur in stage 1 and 2 NREM and REM sleep than in stage 3 or 4 NREM sleep. Events are usually longer and associated with more severe decreases in oxygen saturation when they occur in REM sleep. Snoring between apneas is typically reported by bed partners, as are witnessed episodes of gasping or choking and frequent movements that disrupt sleep. Most patients awaken in the morning feeling tired and unrefreshed regardless of the duration of their time in bed. Excessive sleepiness is a major presenting complaint. The sleepiness is most evident when the patient is in a relaxing inactive situation. The patient's quality of life is adversely affected by unrefreshing sleep, sleepiness, and fatigue and by the disruption of the bed partner's sleep and his or her resultant irritability.

Associated Features

Current evidence suggests that OSA is a significant risk factor for development of systemic hypertension, independent of complicating variables such as obesity. OSA is also associated with type II diabetes, but the nature of the relationship is not well understood. Patients with severe disease may be at risk for developing pulmonary hypertension and cor pulmonale, although this is usually seen only in patients who have comorbid conditions such as morbid obesity or chronic obstructive pulmonary disease. When OSA coexists with dilated cardiomyopathy or ischemic heart disease, there may be worsening of the underlying heart disease and predisposition to congestive heart failure. It is possible for any severity level of OSA to occur with any degree of symptomatic sleepiness and, in some cases, with no subjective complaints. It is important to note that sleepiness is a condition with a multifactorial etiology and a range of manifestations. Different measures of sleepiness, including self-reported severity of sleepiness, commonly used indexes such as the Epworth Sleepiness Scale, and sleepiness measured objectively by the MSLT, are not strongly correlated and, thus, assessment of sleepiness is fraught with potential variability. In addition, patients may adapt to any level of sleepiness over time and fail to view it as a reportable problem.

Demographics

When OSA was defined as an AHI greater than five with a complaint of excessive daytime sleepiness, the prevalence was estimated to be 4% in men and 2% in women. The steepest prevalence increase is in the transition from middle-aged to older-aged adults. In younger, but not in middle-age groups, OSA has been reported to be more prevalent in African Americans compared with Caucasians. The prevalence of OSA in Asian patients with craniofacial features that predispose them to developing OSA may be high in spite of their having a lower BMI in comparison with Caucasian patients.

Predisposing & Precipitating Factors

The major predisposing factor for OSA is excess body weight. Menopause is a risk factor for this disorder in women, even after adjustment for age and BMI. Smokers may also be at higher risk for having OSA. Various abnormalities of the bony and soft tissue structures of the head and neck may predispose the individual to having OSA.

Familial Patterns

Familial clustering of OSA defined by the AHI has been described.

Polysomnographic & Other Objective Findings

Obstructive apneas are documented during polysomnography when there is a cessation of airflow but ongoing respiratory efforts. Obstructive hypopneas are identified when there is a reduction rather than a cessation of airflow with ongoing respiratory effort. Oxygen saturation typically starts to decline for a variable period of time following the onset of an event (apnea or hypopnea), with the nadir usually occurring once normal breathing resumes. If the baseline oxygen saturation is normal, there may be no discernible drop in oxygen saturation despite a clear drop in inspiratory airflow, increased respiratory effort, and a brief change in sleep state (arousal). These events have been defined as RERAs.

The UARS is a proposed diagnostic classification for patients with RERAs who do not also have events that would meet definitions for apneas or hypopneas. However, these events are presumed to have the same underlying pathophysiology as obstructive apneas and hypopneas (upper airway obstruction) and are believed to be as much of a risk factor for symptoms of unrefreshing sleep, daytime somnolence, and fatigue as frank apnea or hypopnea. Therefore, it is recommended that they be included as part of OSA and not considered a separate entity. The EEG may provide evidence of a brief arousal from sleep, and the submental electromyogram may demonstrate a burst of activity indicating upper-airway dilating muscle activation immediately preceding the resumption of normal breathing. Obstructive apneas and hypopneas may be accompanied by bradyarrhythmias, tachyarrhythmias, or both; however, the prevalence of this finding in patients varies widely.

Unresolved Issues & Further Directions
Measurement and definitions of hypopnea events in OSA can vary widely, compromising the usefulness of the AHI cutpoints for diagnosis and research.

Differential Diagnosis
- Patients who have loud disruptive *snoring* as their presenting complaint may only have periods of increased upper airway resistance without documented apneas or hypopneas.
- Patients will sometimes present with symptoms of sudden nocturnal awakenings with a sensation of an inability to breathe. This is an occasional presenting symptom of OSA, but other disorders can produce similar symptoms, including *panic attacks, laryngospasm related to gastroesophageal reflux,* and *dyspnea caused by pulmonary edema.*
- *CSA* can be differentiated from OSA by the lack of chest or abdominal wall movement associated with the central apneas. Mixed apneas may be seen and are included in the diagnosis of OSA.
- OSA must be distinguished from *nonobstructive alveolar hypoventilation.* Adults with lung or chest wall disease may have desaturation and hypercapnia during sleep. It may be difficult to distinguish nonobstructive hypoventilation and desaturation from OSA, especially because the two conditions may coexist. In general, patients with pure nonobstructive hypoventilation will not snore. Oxygen desaturations associated with nonobstructive alveolar hypoventilation are more sustained than those observed in OSA.
- OSA must be differentiated from other causes of sleepiness such as *narcolepsy, idiopathic hypersomnia, insufficient sleep,* and *PLMD.*

Obstructive Sleep Apnea, Pediatric
Please see the Pediatric section of the Manual for this diagnosis.

SLEEP RELATED HYPOVENTILATION/HYPOXEMIC SYNDROMES

Diagnostic Criteria for

Sleep Related Nonobstructive Alveolar Hypoventilation, Idiopathic 327.24

A. Polysomnographic monitoring demonstrates episodes of shallow breathing longer than 10 seconds in duration associated with arterial oxygen desaturation and frequent arousals from sleep associated with the breathing disturbances or brady-tachycardia.

Note: *Although symptoms are not mandatory to make this diagnosis, patients often report excessive daytime sleepiness, frequent arousals and awakenings during sleep, or insomnia complaints.*

B. No primary lung diseases, skeletal malformations, or peripheral neuromuscular disorders that affect ventilation are present.

C. The disorder is not better explained by another current sleep disorder, medical or neurological disorder, mental disorder, medication use, or substance use disorder.

Alternate Names

primary alveolar hypoventilation, idiopathic central alveolar hypoventilation

Essential Features

Sleep related nonobstructive alveolar hypoventilation is characterized by decreased alveolar ventilation resulting in sleep related arterial oxygen desaturation in patients with normal mechanical properties of the lung. In the absence of peripheral impairments, such as severe obesity or abnormalities in pulmonary mechanics such as kyphoscoliosis, the chronic disorder is referred to as *idiopathic central alveolar hypoventilation syndrome*. When the patient presents with diurnal, as well as nocturnal, hypoventilation without a readily identifiable pulmonary, endocrine, neurological, ventilatory, muscle, or cardiac cause, the condition should be referred to as *idiopathic (primary) alveolar hypoventilation*. The defining characteristic is blunted chemoresponsiveness with no other identifiable abnormalities. A consistent feature of idiopathic diurnal hypoventilation is sleep related hypoventilation. Typically, sleep related hypoventilation develops in the early stages of the condition, as a result of removal of the wakefulness stimulus to breathe. The main feature of the condition is reduced ventilation secondary to decreased tidal volume, with ensuing hypercapnia and hypoxemia. Subsequent sleep fragmentation manifests as an ascent to a lighter sleep stage, transient arousals, or awakening. These sleep effects may lead to insomnia or, if the arousals and awakenings are frequent enough, excessive sleepiness. The presenting clinical picture typically includes both features of the underlying ventilatory insufficiency (e.g., morning headache, cor pulmonale, peripheral edema, polycythemia, and abnormal pulmonary function tests) and features of sleep disturbance (e.g., poor nocturnal sleep and daytime sleepiness).

Associated Features

OSA and CSA may coexist with the hypoventilation but are not an intrinsic feature of the condition. In adults, there may be impaired psychosocial or work functioning. Frequent episodes of shallow breathing may be noted to occur during sleep. The clinical signs of hypoxia can be quite subtle in children, who may not look distressed. Children do not develop inspiratory retractions, nasal flaring, or other signs of increased respiratory effort in response to the hypoxia. As a result, hypoxia may progress for quite some time without notice until the child appears to deteriorate suddenly, with cardiopulmonary arrest or severe decompensation.

Polysomnographic & Other Objective Findings

Periods of decreased tidal volume lasting up to several minutes, with sustained arterial oxygen desaturation, are usually observed. These episodes are often worse during REM sleep. OSA may also contribute to the arterial oxygen desaturation but is not the primary cause. Carbon dioxide levels show an increase during the episodes of hypoventilation, with some improvement following the termination of the respiratory event. Patients with normal awake pulmonary function tests may demonstrate a marked decrease in chemoresponsiveness to carbon dioxide. Daytime arterial blood gases may be normal or impaired. Brain imaging may be necessary to detect structural lesions that can account for the impaired respiratory control. No associated lesions are present in the idiopathic form of alveolar hypoventilation syndrome. Rarely, phrenic nerve conduction tests and electromyography, or muscle biopsy of the respiratory musculature, may be indicated. Electrocardiography, chest radiography, and echocardiography may show evidence of pulmonary hypertension. Elevated hematocrit and hemoglobin levels indicate polycythemia from chronic hypoxia.

Differential Diagnosis
- The differential diagnosis of sleep related hypoventilation/hypoxemia includes any disorder that can result in hypoxemia during sleep. Idiopathic sleep related nonobstructive alveolar hypoventilation must be distinguished from other forms of *hypoventilation due to peripheral neurological, muscular, skeletal, orthopedic,* or *pulmonary pathology.*
- *OSA* and *CSA* are distinguished from sleep related hypoventilation/hypoxemia by clinical features and by the presence of periodic alterations in flow, which are typically associated with corresponding periodic alterations in oxygen saturation. Oxygen desaturations associated with sleep related nonobstructive alveolar hypoventilation, idiopathic type, are more sustained, usually several minutes or longer in duration.
- *Cardiac disease* and *hypothyroidism* should also be considered in the differential diagnosis.

Congenital Central Alveolar Hypoventilation
Please see the Pediatric section of the Manual for this diagnosis

Diagnostic Criteria for

Sleep Related Hypoventilation/Hypoxemia Due to Pulmonary Parenchymal or Vascular Pathology 327.26

A. Lung parenchymal disease or pulmonary vascular disease is present and believed to be the primary cause of hypoxemia.

B. Polysomnography or sleeping arterial blood gas determination shows at least one of the following:

    i. An SpO_2 during sleep of less than 90% for more than five minutes with a nadir of at least 85%

    ii. More than 30% of total sleep time at an SpO_2 of less than 90%

    iii. Sleeping arterial blood gas with $PaCO_2$ that is abnormally high or disproportionately increased relative to levels during wakefulness

C. The disorder is not better explained by another current sleep disorder, medical or neurological disorder, medication use, or substance use disorder.

Essential Features

Significant sleep related hypoxemia and the presence of lung parenchymal disease (as documented by pulmonary function testing or radiographic imaging) or pulmonary vascular pathology (as documented by echocardiography, pulmonary artery catheter measurements, or laboratory studies [e.g., in the case of hemoglobinopathies]) are essential features. The observed hypoxemia is not entirely a function of other sleep related breathing disorders such as OSA, CSA or Cheyne Stokes breathing pattern. Diseases known to cause sleep related hypoventilation/hypoxemia due to pulmonary parenchymal or vascular pathology include, but are not limited to, interstitial lung diseases such as desquamative interstitial pneumonitis, usual interstitial pneumonitis, and hypersensitivity pneumonitis; idiopathic and secondary forms of pulmonary hypertension; and sickle cell anemia and other hemoglobinopathies.

The gold standard for identifying sleep related hypoventilation/hypoxemia due to underlying pulmonary parenchymal disease or vascular pathology is sustained (i.e., without saw tooth pattern fluctuations) oxyhemoglobin desaturation in the absence of obstructive, mixed or central apneas or hypopneas, inspiratory airflow limitation (consistent with partial upper airway obstruction), or snoring.

Associated Features
Patients with sleep related hypoventilation/hypoxemia due to pulmonary parenchymal or vascular pathology are at risk for developing the consequences of nocturnal hypoxemia, including pulmonary artery hypertension, cor pulmonale, and neurocognitive dysfunction. Although there is no physiologic link between pulmonary parenchymal or vascular pathology and OSA, these conditions may overlap by chance due to the prevalent nature of OSA.

Predisposing & Precipitating Factors
There is no recognized threshold of pulmonary parenchymal or vascular disease severity that adequately predicts the risk of sleep related hypoventilation/hypoxemia in individual patients. Similarly, the relationship between awake oxyhemoglobin saturation and sleep related desaturation, as well as the relationship between awake arterial $PaCO_2$ and sleep related desaturation, is not sufficiently strong to have substantial predictive value in individual patients. However, it is evident that the greater the perturbation of pulmonary function and vascular involvement and the lower the awake oxyhemoglobin saturation, the greater the risk for sleep related hypoventilation/hypoxemia.

Polysomnographic & Other Objective Findings
The characteristic polysomnographic finding is sustained oxygen desaturation during sleep that is unexplained by discrete apnea and hypopnea events. Intermittent arousal associated with hypoxemia may be observed. The diagnosis may be suggested by overnight oximetry. Typically, in the absence of OSA, CSA, and Cheyne Stokes breathing pattern, desaturations are prolonged and without frequent variation. However, there are no criteria that clearly define these differences.

Differential Diagnosis

- The differential diagnosis of sleep related hypoventilation/hypoxemia includes any disorder that can result in hypoxemia during sleep. Sleep related hypoxemia due to pulmonary parenchymal or vascular pathology must be distinguished from other forms of *hypoventilation due to peripheral neurological, muscular, skeletal,* or *orthopedic lesions.*
- *OSA* and *CSA* are distinguished from sleep related hypoventilation/hypoxemia by clinical features and by the presence of periodic alterations in flow, which are typically associated with corresponding periodic alterations in oxygen saturation.

Diagnostic Criteria for

Sleep Related Hypoventilation/Hypoxemia Due to Lower Airways Obstruction 327.26

A. Lower airways obstructive disease is present (as evidenced by a forced expiratory volume exhaled in one-second/forced vital capacity ratio less than 70% of predicted values on pulmonary function testing) and is believed to be the primary cause of hypoxemia.

B. Polysomnography or sleeping arterial blood gas determination shows at least one of the following:

    i. An SpO_2 during sleep of less than 90% for more than five minutes with a nadir of at least 85%

    ii. More than 30% of total sleep time with an SpO_2 of less than 90%

    iii. Sleeping arterial blood gas with $PaCO_2$ that is abnormally high or disproportionately increased relative to levels during wakefulness

C. The disorder is not better explained by another current sleep disorder, medical or neurological disorder, medication use, or substance use disorder.

Essential Features

Obstruction or increased airflow resistance in airways below the laryngeal apparatus characterizes these disorders. COPD reflects an umbrella term for chronic bronchitis and emphysema. Chronic bronchitis is a clinical entity characterized by a chronic productive cough for at least three months of the year, for at least two consecutive years, in the absence of other identifiable etiologies. Emphysema is further characterized by destruction of lung tissue without evident fibrosis. Emphysema and chronic bronchitis often coexist in patients. Alpha-1 antitrypsin deficiency is a genetic cause of COPD with an incidence of three in 3,000 live births. Bronchiectasis and cystic fibrosis are conditions in which there is obstruction to normal flow of gas. Bronchiectasis is characterized by lower airway inflammation and increased airflow resistance. Increased sputum production is often present as well. Cystic fibrosis was discussed in the section on sleep related hypoventilation/hypoxemia due to pulmonary parenchymal pathology. The gold standard for identifying sleep related hypoventilation/hypoxemia due to lower airways obstruction is a $PaCO_2$ greater than 45 mm Hg measured during sleep. In the absence of arterial blood-gas data, sleep related hypoxemia associated with alveolar hypoventilation may be inferred from prolonged and sustained (i.e., without saw-tooth pattern fluctuations) oxyhemoglobin desaturation in the absence of obstructive, mixed, or central apnea or hypopneas; inspiratory airflow limitation (consistent with partial upper airway obstruction); or snoring. Patients with chronic lower airways obstruction are increasingly predisposed to developing hypoventilation/hypoxemia as the severity of the underlying lower airways obstruction (as reflected by pulmonary function testing) increases.

Associated Features
Patients with sleep related hypoventilation/hypoxemia due to lower airways obstruction are at risk for developing the consequences of nocturnal hypoxemia, including pulmonary artery hypertension, cor pulmonale, and neurocognitive dysfunction. Although there is no physiological link between chronic lower airways obstruction and OSA, both are prevalent disorders and not uncommonly overlap.

Predisposing & Precipitating Factors
There is no recognized threshold of pulmonary parenchymal disease severity that adequately predicts the risk of sleep related hypoventilation/hypoxemia in individual patients. Similarly, the relationship between awake oxyhemoglobin saturation and sleep related desaturation, as well as the relationship between awake $PaCO_2$ and sleep related desaturation, is not sufficiently strong to have substantial predictive value in individual patients. However, it is evident that the greater the perturbation of pulmonary function and the lower the awake oxyhemoglobin saturation, the greater the risk for having sleep related hypoventilation/hypoxemia.

Polysomnographic & Other Objective Findings

The characteristic polysomnographic finding is sustained oxygen desaturation during sleep that is unexplained by discrete apnea and hypopnea events.

Differential Diagnosis

- The differential diagnosis of sleep related hypoventilation/hypoxemia includes any disorder that can result in hypoxemia during sleep. Sleep related hypoventilation/hypoxemia due to lower airways obstruction must be distinguished from other forms of *hypoventilation due to peripheral neurological, muscular, skeletal,* or *orthopedic lesions.*
- *OSA* and *CSA* are distinguished from sleep related hypoventilation/hypoxemia by clinical features and by the presence of periodic alterations in flow, which are typically associated with corresponding periodic alterations in oxygen saturation.

Diagnostic Criteria for

Sleep Related Hypoventilation/Hypoxemia Due to Neuromuscular and Chest Wall Disorders 327.26

A. A neuromuscular or chest wall disorder is present and believed to be the primary cause of hypoxemia.

B. Polysomnography or sleeping arterial blood gas determination shows at least one of the following:

    i. An SpO_2 during sleep of less than 90% for more than five minutes with a nadir of at least 85%

    ii. More than 30% of total sleep time at an SpO_2 of less than 90%

    iii. Sleeping arterial blood gas with $PaCO_2$ that is abnormally high or disproportionately increased relative to levels during wakefulness

C. The disorder is not better explained by another current sleep disorder, medical or neurological disorder, medication use, or substance use disorder.

Alternate Names

obesity-hypoventilation syndrome.

Essential Features

Those neuromuscular and chest wall disorders that are relevant to sleep related alveolar hypoventilation share the common feature of an abnormal "ventilatory pump." Under the conditions imposed by normal sleep physiology, the abnormal pump is unable to meet the ventilatory requirements for maintaining the $PaCO_2$ at or below 45 mm Hg. Impairment of the ventilatory pump in these disorders is related to reduced ventilatory muscle (intercostal, diaphragm, and accessory muscle) contractility or anatomic distortion of the chest wall structures that alters the mechanics and configuration of the ventilatory muscles such that their efficiency is reduced. OSA may coexist with neuromuscular and chest wall disorders. Sleep related hypoventilation/hypoxemia due to neuromuscular and chest wall disorders may be accentuated in the presence of OSA. In addition, some of these patients have reduced central neural chemoresponsiveness. These factors accentuate the impact of abnormal ventilatory muscles on sleep related hypoventilation/hypoxemia due to neuromuscular and chest wall disorders. Obesity predisposes individuals to developing this condition by increasing the burden on disadvantaged ventilatory muscles. Patients with neuromuscular and chest wall disorders are predisposed to developing atelectasis. Atelectasis reduces oxygen stores and predisposes the individual to having oxyhemoglobin desaturation during sleep. In addition, some patients experience abnormal deglutition and increased risk for aspiration of oral contents into the lungs, which also will promote desaturation during sleep.

Associated Features

Patients with sleep related hypoventilation/hypoxemia due to neuromuscular and chest wall disorders are at risk for developing the consequences of nocturnal hypoxemia, including pulmonary artery hypertension, cor pulmonale, and neurocognitive dysfunction.

Predisposing & Precipitating Factors

Patients with hypoxemia during wakefulness are at particular risk for having sleep related hypoxemia. Thus, one of the best predictors of sleep related hypoxemia is reduced awake oxyhemoglobin saturation. Unfortunately, there is substantial variability in the relationship between awake saturation and desaturation during sleep so that the predictive value is very limited in individual patients. Although sleep related hypoventilation/hypoxemia is associated with greater degrees of obesity (and reduced lung volumes and reduced awake oxyhemoglobin saturation), the predictive value of the magnitude of obesity and sleep related hypoventilation/hypoxemia is not sufficiently strong to be very useful in predicting what will occur during sleep in individual patients.

Polysomnographic & Other Objective Findings

Polysomnography demonstrates frequent arousals, increased wakefulness after sleep onset, and reduced amounts of REM sleep. When present, obstructive and central apneas will disrupt sleep and accentuate sleep related oxyhemoglobin desaturation. To the extent that sleep related hypoventilation/hypoxemia due to neuromuscular and chest wall disorders are associated with hypoxemia, such findings as dysrhythmias, arrhythmias, and seizures may be observed during sleep. Due to diaphragm weakness, patients may have orthopnea.

Differential Diagnosis

- The differential diagnosis of sleep related hypoventilation/hypoxemia includes any disorder that can result in hypoxemia during sleep. Sleep related hypoventilation/hypoxemia due to neuromuscular and chest wall disorders must be distinguished from other forms of *hypoventilation due to peripheral neurological or primary pulmonary pathology.*
- *OSA* and *CSA* are distinguished from sleep related hypoventilation/hypoxemia by clinical features and by the presence of periodic alterations in flow, which are typically associated with corresponding periodic alterations in oxygen saturation. Oxygen desaturations associated with sleep related hypoventilation/hypoxemia due to lower airways obstruction are more sustained, usually several minutes or longer in duration.

Other Sleep Related Breathing Disorders 327.20

This diagnosis is used for forms of SRBD that cannot be classified elsewhere or may not neatly fit into one category but are believed to be a function of respiratory disturbance in sleep. In some cases, this diagnosis may be assigned on a temporary basis when an SRBD diagnosis seems appropriate but further evaluation is required to determine the specific type of breathing abnormality in sleep.

III. HYPERSOMNIAS
OF CENTRAL ORIGIN NOT DUE TO A CIRCADIAN RHYTHM SLEEP DISORDER, SLEEP RELATED BREATHING DISORDER, OR OTHER CAUSE OF DISTURBED NOCTURNAL SLEEP

This section includes disorders in which the primary complaint is daytime sleepiness and in which the cause of the primary symptom is not disturbed nocturnal sleep or misaligned circadian rhythms. Daytime sleepiness is defined as the inability to stay awake and alert during the major waking episodes of the day, resulting in unintended lapses into drowsiness or sleep. The severity of daytime sleepiness can be quantified subjectively using severity scales such as the Epworth Sleepiness Scale and objectively using the MSLT and the MWT. These measures are poorly correlated with each other and must be used with appropriate clinical judgment. The MSLT has not been validated as a diagnostic test in children younger than eight years of age.

The MSLT measures the physiological tendency to fall asleep in quiet situations. A mean sleep latency below five minutes has generally been considered as indicative of sleepiness whereas a latency over 10 minutes has generally been considered indicative of normal alertness. In this section, a mean MSLT sleep latency below eight minutes is used to document sleepiness for diagnostic purposes. Of note, the presence of multiple sleep-onset REM periods (SOREMPs) during the MSLT is a much more specific finding in narcolepsy than a mean sleep latency less than or equal to eight minutes, although SOREMPs also can occur in a small number of normal adults and in patients with other sleep disorders, such as SRBDs.

The MWT measures a person's ability to maintain wakefulness in quiet situations. It is primarily used following the treatment of hypersomnia with stimulant medications to objectively document the ability to stay awake.

For the correct interpretation of polysomnographic findings, the recordings should be performed with the following conditions: the patient must be free of drugs that influence sleep for at least 15 days (or at least five times the half-life of the drug and longest-acting metabolite); the sleep-wake schedule must have been standardized for at least seven days before the polysomnographic testing (and documented by sleep log or actigraphy); and nocturnal polysomnography should be performed on the night immediately preceding the MSLT to rule out other sleep disorders. The MSLT may be difficult to interpret if the patient did not sleep a sufficient number of hours during nocturnal polysomnography (a minimum of six hours is expected but some patients may require more).

In all cases in which a diagnosis of hypersomnia is to be made, a review of psychiatric history and drug and medication use and an assessment of other sleep and medical disorders should be performed.

Clinically significant associated SRBDs or PLMS during sleep may be present and, if so, should be treated prior to diagnosing many of these conditions.

Diagnostic Criteria for

Narcolepsy With Cataplexy 347.01

A. The patient has a complaint of excessive daytime sleepiness occurring almost daily for at least three months.

B. A definite history of cataplexy, defined as sudden and transient episodes of loss of muscle tone triggered by emotions, is present.

Note: To be labeled as cataplexy, these episodes must be triggered by strong emotions—most reliably laughing or joking—and must be generally bilateral and brief (less than two minutes). Consciousness is preserved, at least at the beginning of the episode. Observed cataplexy with transient reversible loss of deep tendon reflexes is a very strong, but rare, diagnostic finding.

C. The diagnosis of narcolepsy with cataplexy should, whenever possible, be confirmed by nocturnal polysomnography followed by an MSLT; the mean sleep latency on MSLT is less than or equal to eight minutes and two or more SOREMPs are observed following sufficient nocturnal sleep (minimum six hours) during the night prior to the test. Alternatively, hypocretin-1 levels in the CSF are less than or equal to 110 pg/mL or one-third of mean normal control values.

Note: The presence of two or more SOREMPs during the MSLT is a very specific finding, whereas a mean sleep latency of less than eight minutes can be found in up to 30% of the normal population. Low CSF hypocretin-1 levels (less than or equal to 110 pg/mL or one-third of mean normal control values) are found in more than 90% of patients with narcolepsy with cataplexy and almost never in controls or in other patients with other pathologies.

D. The hypersomnia is not better explained by another sleep disorder, medical or neurological disorder, mental disorder, medication use, or substance use disorder.

Alternate Names

Gélineau syndrome.

Essential Features

Narcolepsy with cataplexy is primarily characterized by excessive daytime sleepiness and cataplexy. Many of the symptoms of narcolepsy with cataplexy are due to an unusual proclivity to transition rapidly from wakefulness into REM sleep and to experience dissociated REM sleep events. Narcolepsy with cataplexy affects 0.02% to 0.18% of the United States and Western European population. Onset almost always occurs after five years of age, most typically between ages 15 and 25. Excessive daytime sleepiness is usually the most disabling symptom and is often the first to occur. It is characterized by repeated naps or lapses into sleep during monotonous situations such as while watching television. Patients with narcolepsy with cataplexy typically nap for a short duration and awaken refreshed but within two or three hours begin to feel sleepy again. Sudden and often irresistible sleep attacks (a sudden onset of sleep or involuntary sleep episodes) may also occur in unusual situations such as eating, walking, or driving within a background of overall sleepiness. When sleepiness is severe, a symptom called "automatic behavior" is occasionally observed: the patient continues an activity in a semiautomatic fashion without memory or consciousness. Cataplexy, a unique symptom of narcolepsy, is characterized by sudden and bilateral loss of muscle tone provoked by strong emotions. These triggering emotions are usually positive (e.g., laughter, pride, elation, or surprise) but are sometimes negative (e.g., anger). Cataplexy can include all skeletal muscle groups or it can be localized. The duration of cataplexy is usually short, ranging from a few seconds to several minutes at most, and recovery is immediate and complete. The loss of muscle tone ranges from a mild sensation of weakness—with head drop, facial sagging, jaw weakness, slurred speech, or buckling of the knees—to complete postural collapse. Twitches and jerks may occur, particularly in the face, as the patient is trying to fight the episode. Serious injury from cataplexy is rare because it usually takes several seconds for weakness to fully develop. The frequency of cataplexy shows wide interpersonal variation from rare events during a year-long period in some patients to countless attacks in a single day in others. Strong emotions or abrupt withdrawal from adrenergic or serotonergic antidepressant medications may provoke successive episodes of cataplexy, termed *status cataplecticus*.

Current evidence suggests that most cases of narcolepsy with cataplexy are associated with the loss of approximately 50,000 to 100,000 hypothalamic neurons containing the neuropeptide hypocretin, also called orexin. The lack of hypocretin can be best assessed by measuring CSF hypocretin-1 (orexin-A). Approximately 90% of patients with narcolepsy with cataplexy, almost all with HLA DQB1*0602, have dramatically decreased CSF levels.

Because narcolepsy with cataplexy is HLA associated, it is hypothesized that the cause of most cases is an autoimmune destruction of hypocretin cells that generally occurs during adolescence.

Associated Features

Sleep paralysis, hypnagogic hallucinations, and nocturnal sleep disruption commonly occur in patients with narcolepsy with cataplexy. However, these symptoms also occasionally occur in normal people and in patients with other sleep disorders. Hypnagogic hallucinations are vivid perceptual experiences typically occurring at sleep onset, often with realistic awareness of the presence of someone or something, and include visual, tactile, kinetic, and auditory phenomena. The accompanying affect is often fear or dread. Sleep paralysis is a transient, generalized inability to move or to speak during the transition between sleep and wakefulness. The patient usually regains muscular control within several minutes. Sleep paralysis is a frightening experience, particularly when initially experienced, and often is accompanied by a sensation of an inability to breathe. Forty percent to 80% of narcoleptic patients have sleep paralysis or hypnagogic hallucinations. Nocturnal sleep disruption occurs in approximately 50% of narcoleptics and can even be the presenting symptom. It is often a very disabling symptom that may exacerbate all other symptoms. Narcoleptic patients may report memory lapses, ptosis, blurred vision, and diplopia, most likely because of sleepiness. RBD is also observed at a greater-than-expected frequency in patients with narcolepsy with cataplexy. It can be either an isolated polysomnographic finding (subclinical RBD) or a clinically significant complaint that may require specific treatment. Narcolepsy with cataplexy is often associated with increased BMI and, more rarely, obesity, especially when untreated. This increased BMI may predispose the individual to develop OSA.

Polysomnographic & Other Objective Findings

Narcolepsy with cataplexy can be diagnosed on purely clinical grounds, but additional tests are useful to confirm the diagnosis. Most commonly, nocturnal polysomnography followed by the MSLT is recommended to assess the severity of sleepiness and diagnose other concomitant sleep disorders. All-night polysomnography frequently shows a short sleep latency of less than 10 minutes and a short REM sleep latency. Stage 1 sleep and the number of awakenings may be increased. The MSLT demonstrates a mean latency of less than eight minutes, typically less than five minutes, and two or more SOREMPs. Approximately 15% of patients with narcolepsy with cataplexy, especially patients older than 36 years of age, may have normal or borderline MSLT results. Typing for HLA almost always shows the presence of HLA DQB1*0602 (and DR2 or DRB1*1501 in Caucasians and Asians), but this is not diagnostic for narcolepsy. Typing is most useful to exclude a diagnosis of narcolepsy with cataplexy in selected cases. Measuring CSF levels of hypocretin-1 is highly specific and sensitive for the diagnosis of narcolepsy with cataplexy. Values below 110 pg/mL (30% of mean control value) are found in about 90% of patients with narcolepsy with cataplexy, though CSF hypocretin assays are not yet standardized across labs. Low CSF hypocretin values are occasionally observed in seriously ill patients with other disorders and should be interpreted within the clinical context.

Clinical & Pathophysiological Subtypes

In general, the risk of a first-degree relative developing narcolepsy with cataplexy is only 1% to 2%, but rare families have more than two members with narcolepsy with cataplexy.

Differential Diagnosis

- Narcolepsy with cataplexy is differentiated from *narcolepsy without cataplexy* by the presence of definite cataplexy.
- *Idiopathic hypersomnia* lacks cataplexy and two or more SOREMPS on MSLT.
- *Recurrent hypersomnia* can produce excessive sleepiness, but patients sleep normally between episodes.
- Cataplexy should be differentiated from *hypotension, transient ischemic attacks, drop attacks, akinetic seizures, neuromuscular disorders, vestibular disorders, psychological or psychiatric disorders,* and *sleep paralysis.*
- Excessive daytime sleepiness may result from *OSA, PLMD, environmental sleep disorder,* or *behaviorally induced insufficient sleep syndrome*
- *Pseudonarcolepsy and pseudocataplexy* are equivalents of a conversion disorder.

Pediatrics

The daytime sleepiness of narcolepsy may present as sleeping at school or the reappearance of regular daytime naps. Narcolepsy in children can also manifest as behavioral problems, decreased performance, inattentiveness, lack of energy, or insomnia. Affected children may be misdiagnosed with attention-deficit/hyperactivity disorder, schizophrenia, or depression. Episodes of cataplexy may be misdiagnosed as seizures. The presence of sleep paralysis or hypnagogic hallucinations may be difficult to confirm, depending on the child's verbal ability. Narcolepsy with cataplexy is extremely rare prior to the age of four years.

Diagnostic Criteria for

Narcolepsy Without Cataplexy 347.00

A. The patient has a complaint of excessive daytime sleepiness occurring almost daily for at least three months.

B. Typical cataplexy is not present, although doubtful or atypical cataplexy-like episodes may be reported.

C. The diagnosis of narcolepsy without cataplexy must be confirmed by nocturnal polysomnography followed by an MSLT. In narcolepsy without cataplexy, the mean sleep latency on MSLT is less than or equal to eight minutes and two or more SOREMPs are observed following sufficient nocturnal sleep (minimum six hours) during the night prior to the test.

Note: *The presence of two or more SOREMPs during the MSLT is a specific finding, whereas a mean sleep latency of less than eight minutes can be found in up to 30% of the normal population.*

D. The hypersomnia is not better explained by another sleep disorder, medical or neurological disorder, mental disorder, medication use, or substance use disorder.

Essential Features

Excessive daytime sleepiness in narcolepsy without cataplexy is most typically associated with naps that are refreshing in nature while nocturnal sleep is normal or moderately disturbed without excessive amounts of sleep. Sleep paralysis, hypnagogic hallucinations, or automatic behavior may be present. The MSLT demonstrates a mean sleep latency less than or equal to eight minutes and two or more SOREMPs. Measuring CSF hypocretin-1 is highly specific and sensitive for the diagnosis of narcolepsy with cataplexy. In contrast, values below 110 pg/ml (one-third of mean control value) are highly specific but are only rarely observed in cases of narcolepsy without cataplexy. Narcolepsy without cataplexy typically begins during adolescence and may occur in 0.02% of the population.

Associated Features

Some patients have memory lapses, ptosis, blurred vision, and diplopia. Unambiguous cataplexy is absent, but cataplexy-like episodes may be reported. These include atypical sensations of muscle weakness triggered by unusual emotions such as stress, sex or intense activity/exercise; long episodes of tiredness; and episodes that have occurred only a few times in a lifetime. Nightmares and RBD may occur. Nocturnal sleep disruption with frequent awakenings may occur.

Polysomnographic & Other Objective Findings

All-night polysomnography often shows a sleep latency of less than 10 minutes and a SOREMP, and sometimes an increase in stage 1 sleep and the number of awakenings. The MSLT demonstrates a mean sleep latency of less than eight minutes, with two or more SOREMPs. About 40% of patients are HLA DQB1*0602 positive.

Differential Diagnosis

- See section on *narcolepsy with cataplexy.*

Pediatrics

The daytime sleepiness of narcolepsy may present as sleeping at school or the reappearance of regular daytime naps. Narcolepsy in children can also manifest as behavioral problems, decreased performance, inattentiveness, lack of energy, or insomnia. Affected children may be misdiagnosed with attention-deficit/hyperactivity disorder, schizophrenia, or depression. The presence of sleep paralysis or hypnagogic hallucinations may be difficult to confirm, depending on the child's verbal ability. Narcolepsy without cataplexy is extremely rare prior to the age of four years.

In all pediatric cases, one should consider the possibility that the patient will, with time, develop full narcolepsy with cataplexy.

In peri-pubertal children and adolescents, the most common causes of short sleep latencies, often with multiple SOREMPs on the MSLT, are chronic sleep deprivation and delayed sleep phase syndrome.

Diagnostic Criteria for

Narcolepsy Due to Medical Condition (without cataplexy - 347.10) (with cataplexy – 347.11)

A. The patient has a complaint of excessive daytime sleepiness occurring almost daily for at least three months.
B. One of the following must be observed:
   i. A definite history of cataplexy, defined as sudden and transient episodes of loss of muscle tone (muscle weakness) triggered by emotions, is present

Note: To be cataplexy, these episodes must be triggered by strong emotions, most reliably laughing or joking, and must be generally bilateral and brief (less than two minutes). Consciousness is preserved at least at the beginning of the episode. In narcolepsy (with cataplexy) due to a medical condition, the diagnosis should, whenever possible, be confirmed by nocturnal polysomnography followed by an MSLT (see MSLT criteria below).

   ii. If cataplexy is not present or is very atypical, polysomnographic monitoring performed over the patient's habitual sleep period followed by an MSLT must demonstrate a mean sleep latency on the MSLT of less than eight minutes with two or more SOREMPs, despite sufficient nocturnal sleep prior to the test (minimum six hours)

Note: The presence of two or more SOREMPs during the MSLT is a very specific finding, whereas a mean sleep latency of less than eight minutes can be found in up to 30% of the general population.

   iii. Hypocretin-1 levels in the CSF are less than 110 pg/mL (or 30% of normal control values), provided the patient is not comatose

Note: In patients with severe medical or neurological illness, nocturnal polysomnography or the MSLT may be impossible to conduct or to interpret. Similarly, the value of measuring hypocretin-1 levels in the CSF in critically ill patients is uncertain. Abnormal polysomnography and low CSF hypocretin-1 levels should be interpreted within the clinical context.

C. A significant underlying medical or neurological disorder accounts for the daytime sleepiness
D. The hypersomnia is not better explained by another sleep disorder, mental disorder, medication use, or substance use disorder.

Alternate Names

Secondary narcolepsy, symptomatic narcolepsy.

Essential Features

The direct cause of narcolepsy due to medical condition is a coexisting medical or neurological disorder. Narcolepsy must be documented either clinically (with definite cataplexy), or polysomnographically (a short mean sleep latency and two SOREMPs on the MSLT). All these patients have daytime sleepiness, and some have sleep paralysis, hypnagogic hallucinations, or insomnia. Disorders reported to produce narcolepsy with cataplexy include lesions of the hypothalamus, tumors, strokes, sarcoidosis, paraneoplastic encephalitis (anti-Ma2 antibodies), Neimann-Pick type C disease, and Coffin-Lowry Syndrome. Several other neurological disorders have been associated with narcolepsy, generally without cataplexy, including head trauma, multiple sclerosis, myotonic dystrophy, Prader-Willi syndrome, Parkinson's disease, and multiple system atrophy. In complex cases, for example, after head trauma, clinical judgment should be used to determine if the development of narcolepsy was a mere coincidence or was triggered by the event. In disorders associated with SRBDs (e.g., myotonic dystrophy or Prader-Willi syndrome), this diagnostic category should be used only if SOREMPs on the MSLT persist after the SRBD is adequately treated.

Polysomnographic & Other Objective Findings

Nocturnal polysomnography may show normal or moderately disturbed sleep. In cases without cataplexy, the MSLT must show a mean sleep latency less than eight minutes and two or more SOREMPs. Unless the patient is comatose, CSF hypocretin-1 levels less than 110 pg/mL are a sufficient alternative to the MSLT.

Differential Diagnosis

- The major challenge in establishing a diagnosis of narcolepsy due to medical condition is determination of whether the associated medical or neurological disorder is causing the narcolepsy or is merely associated with the condition. *See previous narcolepsy sections for additional differential diagnoses.*

Narcolepsy, Unspecified

This diagnosis is used on a temporary basis when the patient meets clinical and MSLT criteria for narcolepsy, but further evaluation is required to determine the specific diagnostic category for narcolepsy.

Diagnostic Criteria for

Recurrent Hypersomnia (Including Kleine-Levin Syndrome and Menstrual-Related Hypersomnia) 327.13

A. The patient experiences recurrent episodes of excessive sleepiness of two days to four weeks duration.

B. Episodes recur at least once a year.

C. The patient has normal alertness, cognitive functioning and behavior between attacks.

D. The hypersomnia is not better explained by another sleep disorder, medical or neurological disorder, mental disorder, medication use, or substance use disorder.

Alternate Names
Periodic hypersomnia.

Essential Features
The best-characterized recurrent hypersomnia is Kleine-Levin syndrome, and this section primarily pertains to this rare condition. These patients have recurrent episodes of hypersomnia often associated with other symptoms that typically occur weeks or months apart. Episodes usually last a few days to several weeks and appear once to 10 times a year. Episodes are often preceded by prodromes such as fatigue or headache lasting a few hours. Patients may sleep as long as 16 hours to 18 hours per day, waking or getting up only to eat and void. Urinary incontinence does not occur. Body weight gain of a few kilograms is often observed during the episode. Cognitive abnormalities such as feelings of unreality, confusion, and hallucinations may occur. Behavioral abnormalities such as binge eating, hypersexuality, irritability, and aggressiveness may be present. Patients may respond verbally, but often unclearly or aggressively, when aroused by strong stimuli during the episode. The simultaneous occurrence of all these symptoms is the exception rather than the rule, and in some cases, isolated recurrent hypersomnia may be the only symptom. The disorder usually begins in adolescence and is more common in males.

Polysomnographic & Other Objective Findings

Routine EEGs obtained during episodes have shown general slowing of background electroencephalographic activity and paroxysmal bursts of bisynchronous, generalized, moderate- to high-voltage 5- to 7-Hz waves lasting 0.5-2 seconds. Nocturnal polysomnography shows reduced sleep efficiency and increased wake time after sleep onset. Results of the MSLT are highly dependent on the subject's willingness to comply with the procedure. Twenty-four hour polysomnography demonstrates prolonged total sleep time, up to 18 hours or more in some reports.

Clinical & Pathophysiological Subtypes

Kleine-Levin syndrome: A diagnosis of Kleine-Levin syndrome should be reserved for cases in which recurrent episodes of hypersomnia are clearly associated with behavioral abnormalities such as binge eating; hypersexuality; irritability; aggression; and cognitive abnormalities such as feeling of unreality, confusion, and hallucinations.

Menstrual-related hypersomnia: Recurrent episodes of sleepiness that occur in association with the menstrual cycle may be indicative of the menstrual-related hypersomnia. The condition occurs within the first months after menarche. Episodes generally last one week, with rapid resolution at the time of menses. Hormone imbalance is a likely explanation for the hypersomnia, since oral contraceptives will usually lead to prolonged remission.

Differential Diagnosis

- Recurrent waxing and waning episodes of sleepiness may be secondary to *brain tumors, encephalitis, head trauma,* or *stroke.*
- Recurrent episodes of sleepiness are also reported in the context of psychiatric disorders, such as *bipolar disorder, seasonal affective disorder, and somatoform disorder.*
- Other differential diagnoses include excessive sleepiness due to *OSA, narcolepsy, idiopathic hypersomnia, PLMD, behaviorally induced insufficient sleep syndrome, and environmental sleep disorder.* In these disorders, however, the complaint of excessive sleepiness occurs daily and is usually not recurrent or periodic.

Pediatrics

The onset of the condition has been reported in children as young as six years of age. Most cases affect adolescents.

Diagnostic Criteria for

Idiopathic Hypersomnia With Long Sleep Time 327.11

A. The patient has a complaint of excessive daytime sleepiness occurring almost daily for at least three months.

B. The patient has prolonged nocturnal sleep time (more than 10 hours) documented by interview, actigraphy, or sleep logs. Waking up in the morning or at the end of naps is almost always laborious.

C. Nocturnal polysomnography has excluded other causes of daytime sleepiness.

D. The polysomnogram demonstrates a short sleep latency and a major sleep period that is prolonged to more than 10 hours in duration.

E. If an MSLT is performed following overnight polysomnography, a mean sleep latency of less than eight minutes is found and fewer than two SOREMPs are recorded. Mean sleep latency in idiopathic hypersomnia with long sleep time has been shown to be 6.2 ± 3.0 minutes.

Note: *A mean sleep latency on the MSLT of less than eight minutes can be found in up to 30% of the general population. Both the mean sleep latency on the MSLT and the clinician's interpretation of the patient's symptoms, most notably a clinically significant complaint of sleepiness, should be taken into account in reaching the diagnosis of idiopathic hypersomnia with long sleep time.*

F. The hypersomnia is not better explained by another sleep disorder, medical or neurological disorder, mental disorder, medication use, or substance use disorder.

Note: *Of particular importance, head trauma should not be considered to be the cause of the sleepiness.*

Essential Features

Idiopathic hypersomnia with long sleep time is characterized by constant and severe sleepiness with prolonged but unrefreshing naps of up to three or four hours. The major sleep episode is prolonged to at least 10 hours (typically 12 to 14 hours) with few or no awakenings. Post-awakening confusion (sleep drunkenness) and difficulty waking up are common. Symptoms usually begin in young adulthood and persist for many years. This disorder occasionally runs in families.

Associated Features

Associated symptoms suggesting a dysfunction of the autonomic nervous system may be present, including headaches, which may be migrainous in quality; orthostatic hypotension with syncope; and peripheral vascular complaints (Raynaud's-type phenomena with cold hands and feet). Idiopathic hypersomnia with long sleep time has a variable response to stimulants such as amphetamines, methylphenidate, or modafinil.

Polysomnographic & Other Objective Findings

Polysomnographic monitoring generally demonstrates normal sleep of prolonged duration. An increase in slow-wave sleep may be observed. The MSLT should be performed when possible. However, it may be extremely difficult to wake the patient in preparation for the test or to keep the patient awake between naps. Mean sleep latency in patients with idiopathic hypersomnia (with and without long sleep) has been shown to be 6.2 ± 3.0 minutes. Fewer than two SOREMPs are present. In cases with normal MSLT findings, several authors have suggested the use of long-term (24-hour to 36-hour) sleep monitoring to document excessive amounts of sleep (typically more than 11 to 12 hours per 24 hours). A computed tomography scan, magnetic resonance imaging, or both, should be performed if there is a clinical suspicion of an underlying brain lesion. A psychiatric evaluation should also be considered to exclude the possibility of hypersomnia not due to substance or known physiological condition (i.e., secondary to a psychiatric disorder).

Differential Diagnosis

- Idiopathic hypersomnia with long sleep time should be distinguished from *idiopathic hypersomnia without long sleep time*.
- Idiopathic hypersomnia may be confused with *OSA* or *UARS*, and esophageal monitoring should be considered if the patient has recurrent arousals.
- The MSLT usually shows two or more SOREMPs and a short mean sleep latency in *narcolepsy*.
- *Hypersomnia not due to substance or known physiological condition* should be considered in patients with a personality disorder or a psychiatric condition, most typically depression.
- Hypersomnia can also occur with drug or medication abuse or medication use, brain lesions, or head trauma. Other causes include *long sleepers* and *behaviorally induced insufficient sleep syndrome*.

Pediatrics

Idiopathic hypersomnia is rarely seen before adolescence.

Idiopathic Hypersomnia Without Long Sleep Time 327.12

A. The patient has a complaint of excessive daytime sleepiness occurring almost daily for at least three months.

B. The patient has normal nocturnal sleep (greater than six hours but less than 10 hours) documented by interviews, actigraphy, or sleep logs.

C. Nocturnal polysomnography has excluded other causes of daytime sleepiness.

D. Polysomnography demonstrates a major sleep period that is normal in duration (greater than six hours but less than 10 hours).

E. An MSLT following overnight polysomnography demonstrates a mean sleep latency of less than eight minutes and fewer than two SOREMPs. Mean sleep latency in idiopathic hypersomnia has been shown to be 6.2 ± 3.0 minutes.

Note: *A mean sleep latency of less than eight minutes can be found in up to 30% of the general population. Both the mean sleep latency on the MSLT and the clinician's interpretation of the patient's symptoms, most notably a clinically significant complaint of sleepiness, should be taken into account in reaching the diagnosis of idiopathic hypersomnia without long sleep time.*

F. The hypersomnia is not better explained by another sleep disorder, medical or neurological disorder, mental disorder, medication use, or substance use disorder.

Essential Features

The major clinical feature is a complaint of constant and severe excessive daytime sleepiness, with unintended and generally nonrefreshing naps. The major sleep episode (e.g., nighttime) is either normal duration or slightly prolonged (less than 10 hours), usually with few or no awakenings. Cataplexy is absent.

Associated Features

See idiopathic hypersomnia with long sleep time

Polysomnographic & Other Objective Findings

Nocturnal sleep may be slightly prolonged but is less than 10 hours. Nocturnal sleep must be more than six hours. NREM and REM are in normal proportion. Sleep efficiency usually exceeds 85%. An MSLT should be performed whenever possible. The MSLT usually demonstrates a mean sleep latency of less than eight minutes. Fewer than two SOREMPs are present. A computed tomography scan, magnetic resonance imaging, or both, are indicated to rule out a secondary neurological etiology. A psychiatric evaluation should also be considered to exclude the possibility of hypersomnia not due to substance or known physiological condition (i.e., secondary to psychiatric disorder).

Differential Diagnosis
See *idiopathic hypersomnia with long sleep time*.

Diagnostic Criteria for

Behaviorally Induced Insufficient Sleep Syndrome 307.44

A. The patient has a complaint of excessive sleepiness or, in prepubertal children, a complaint of behavioral abnormalities suggesting sleepiness. The abnormal sleep pattern is present almost daily for at least three months.

B. The patient's habitual sleep episode, established using history, a sleep log, or actigraphy, is usually shorter than expected from age-adjusted normative data.

Note: In the case of individuals with long sleep time, habitual sleep periods may be normal, based on age-adjusted normative data. However, these sleep periods may be insufficient for this population.

C. When the habitual sleep schedule is not maintained (weekends or vacation time), patients will sleep considerably longer than usual.

D. When polysomnography is performed, sleep latency is less than 10 minutes and sleep efficiency greater than 90%. During the MSLT, a short mean latency of less than eight minutes (with or without multiple SOREMPs) may be observed.

E. The hypersomnia is not better explained by another sleep disorder, medical or neurological disorder, mental disorder, medication use, or substance use disorder.

Essential Features
Behaviorally induced insufficient sleep syndrome occurs when an individual persistently fails to obtain the amount of sleep required to maintain normal levels of alertness and wakefulness. The individual engages in voluntary, albeit

unintentional, chronic sleep deprivation. Examination reveals unimpaired or above-average ability to initiate and maintain sleep, with little or no psychopathology. A detailed history of the current sleep pattern reveals a substantial disparity between the need for sleep and the amount actually obtained. Its significance is unappreciated by the patient. A markedly extended sleep time on weekend nights or during holidays as compared to weekday nights is also suggestive of this disorder. Insufficient sleep may be more frequent in adolescence, when sleep need is high but social pressure and tendency to delayed sleep phase often lead to chronic restricted sleep. Elimination of symptoms in response to a therapeutic trial of longer sleep time is diagnostic of behaviorally induced insufficient sleep.

Associated Features

Some individuals may develop irritability, concentration and attention deficits, reduced vigilance, distractibility, reduced motivation, anergia, dysphoria, fatigue, restlessness, incoordination, and malaise. Secondary symptoms may become the main focus of the patient, serving to obscure the primary cause of the difficulties. Sleep paralysis and hypnagogic hallucinations may occur.

Polysomnographic & Other Objective Findings

Polysomnographic evaluation reveals reduced sleep latency, high (greater than 90%) sleep efficiency, and a prolonged sleep time when left to sleep ad lib. The distribution of REM and NREM sleep stages is normal. The MSLT reveals excessive sleepiness, with stage 2 sleep in more than 80% of naps. Measures of sleep-onset latency and the disparity between reported sleep at home and observed total sleep time in the sleep laboratory are the most sensitive and specific measures. Polysomnographic monitoring is not initially required to establish a diagnosis of behaviorally induced insufficient sleep syndrome. Rather, sleep time is extended first, and the patient is reevaluated. If a therapeutic trial with a longer sleep episode eliminates the symptoms, behaviorally induced insufficient sleep syndrome is diagnosed.

Differential Diagnosis

- Behaviorally induced insufficient sleep syndrome may be confused with *narcolepsy* or other *hypersomnias* because an abnormal MSLT (even with two SOREMPs) can be observed as the result of acute or chronic sleep deprivation. The confusion may be most frequently encountered in adolescents or young adults.
- The differential diagnosis of behaviorally induced insufficient sleep syndrome includes numerous other conditions that may result in daytime sleepiness or shortening of nocturnal sleep duration. These include *environmental sleep disorder, psychophysiological insomnia, affective disorder, SRBDs, long sleeper or short sleeper, circadian rhythm sleep disorders*, and *PLMD*.

Diagnostic Criteria for

Hypersomnia Due to Medical Condition 327.14

A. The patient has a complaint of excessive sleepiness present almost daily for at least three months.

B. A significant underlying medical or neurological disorder accounts for the daytime sleepiness.

C. If an MSLT is performed, the mean sleep latency is less than eight minutes with no more than one SOREMP following polysomnographic monitoring performed over the patient's habitual sleep period, with a minimum total sleep time of six hours.

D. The hypersomnia is not better explained by another sleep disorder, mental disorder, medication use, or substance use disorder.

Note: In patients with severe medical or neurological illness, conducting and interpreting the results of nocturnal polysomnography or the MSLT may be impossible. Abnormal polysomnographic results should be interpreted within the clinical context. Additionally, mean sleep latency on MSLT of less than eight minutes can be found in up to 30% of the general population. A clinically significant complaint of excessive daytime sleepiness is far more important than is short sleep latency on MSLT in the diagnosis of hypersomnia due to medical condition.

Essential Features

Hypersomnia due to medical condition is caused by a coexisting medical or neurological disorder. Daytime sleepiness varies in severity and may resemble that of either narcolepsy (i.e., refreshing effects of naps) or idiopathic hypersomnia with long sleep time (i.e., a long sleep episode and unrefreshing sleep). Sleep paralysis, hypnagogic hallucinations, or automatic behavior may or may not be present. Features of narcolepsy such as cataplexy or two or more SOREMPs are absent. Hypersomnia can occur with Parkinson's disease, head trauma, genetic disorders (e.g., Prader-Willi syndrome, myotonic dystrophy), and lesions of the hypothalamus or brainstem (tumors, strokes, encephalitis). Medical causes include endocrine disorders (e.g., hypothyroidism, adrenal insufficiency), hepatic encephalopathy, renal insufficiency, or pancreatic insufficiency. Toxins such as methylchloride, trichloroethylene, and organic solvents may also produce hypersomnia. In the case of disorders associated with both SRBDs and hypersomnia due to medical condition, a diagnosis of hypersomnia due to medical condition should be made only if the hypersomnia persists after adequate treatment of the SRBDs.

Polysomnographic & Other Objective Findings

Nocturnal polysomnography may show normal or moderately disturbed sleep. Nocturnal sleep time must be longer than six hours. MSLT usually shows short sleep latencies. There must be no more than one SOREMP.

Differential Diagnosis

- *See the differential diagnosis for previous hypersomnia sections.* The major challenge in establishing a diagnosis of hypersomnia due to medical condition is determination of whether the associated medical or neurological disorder is causing the hypersomnia or is merely associated with the condition.
- If a mean sleep latency shorter than eight minutes and multiple SOREMPs are observed during the MSLT, or cataplexy is present, the patient should be diagnosed as having *narcolepsy due to medical condition.*
- Where appropriate, hypersomnias should be classified as *hypersomnia not due to substance or known physiological condition* or *hypersomnia due to drug or substance.*
- *Hypersomnia secondary to psychiatric disorders, drugs of abuse, or the effects of prescribed medications* are classified elsewhere.

Pediatrics

Special attention should be given to genetic disorders in the pediatric population.

Diagnostic Criteria for

Hypersomnia Due to Drug or Substance (Abuse) 292.85 (for Alcohol use 291.82)

A. The patient has a complaint of sleepiness or excessive sleep.
B. The complaint is believed to be secondary to current use, recent discontinuation, or prior prolonged use of drugs.
C. The hypersomnia is not better explained by another sleep disorder, medical or neurological disorder, mental disorder, or medication use.

Diagnostic Criteria for

Hypersomnia Due to Drug or Substance (Medications) 292.85

A. The patient has a complaint of sleepiness or excessive sleep.
B. The complaint is associated with current use, recent discontinuation, or prior prolonged use of a prescribed medication.
C. The hypersomnia is not better explained by another sleep disorder, medical or neurological disorder, mental disorder, or substance use disorder.

Essential Features

This diagnostic category should be reserved for patients with excessive nocturnal sleep, daytime sleepiness, or excessive napping that is believed to be secondary to substance use. Hypersomnia due to drug or substance covers hypersomnias associated with tolerance to or withdrawal from various prescribed drugs, street drugs, and alcohol. If narcolepsy or hypersomnia existed prior to stimulant abuse, this category should not be used. Abrupt cessation of prescribed or abused stimulants can produce hypersomnia, and in some cases this sleepiness lasts for many years. Hypersomnia or daytime sleepiness may be secondary to sedative use, such as benzodiazepines, barbiturate, gammahydroxybutyric acid, or alcohol. Daytime sleepiness also occurs with antiepileptic medications and opioid analgesics.

Polysomnographic & Other Objective Findings

Polysomnography is not generally required unless a concomitant sleep disorder is suspected. Nocturnal polysomnography and MSLT results may be variable, depending on the specific substance in question and on the timing of the most recent intake.

Differential Diagnosis

- Hypersomnia or daytime sleepiness often occurs in *idiopathic hypersomnia, narcolepsy, SRBDs, PLMS, chronic fatigue syndrome, behaviorally induced insufficient sleep syndrome,* or *environmental sleep disorder.*

Diagnostic Criteria for

Hypersomnia Not Due to Substance or Known Physiological Condition (Nonorganic Hypersomnia, NOS) 327.15

A. The patient has a complaint of excessive daytime sleepiness or excessive sleep.

B. The complaint is temporally associated with a psychiatric diagnosis.

C. Polysomnographic monitoring demonstrates both of the following:
  - i. Reduced sleep efficiency and increased frequency and duration of awakenings
  - ii. Variable, often normal, mean sleep latencies on the MSLT

D. The hypersomnia is not better explained by another sleep disorder, medical or neurological disorder, medication use, or substance use disorder.

Alternate Names

Hypersomnia associated with mental disorders, psychiatric hypersomnia, secondary hypersomnia (psychiatric), sleep hypochondriasis, pseudohypersomnia or pseudonarcolepsy.

Essential Features

In hypersomnia not due to substance or known physiological condition, excessive nocturnal sleep, daytime sleepiness, or excessive napping are reported; sleep is perceived as nonrestorative and generally of poor quality. Patients are often intensely focused on their hypersomnia, and psychiatric symptoms typically become apparent only after prolonged interviews or psychometric testing. Causative psychiatric conditions include mood disorders, conversion or undifferentiated somatoform disorder, and less frequently other mental disorders such as schizoaffective disorder, adjustment disorder, or personality disorders. This disorder accounts for 5% to 7% of hypersomnia cases and appears more common in women between 20 and 50 years. Poor work attendance, spending full days in bed once or twice a week or abruptly leaving work because of a perceived need to sleep, are common. The hypersomnia is typically associated with lack of interest and social withdrawal. Energy level is decreased, and there is a tendency to spend long hours in bed without sleeping deeply, rather than a true increase in sleep propensity.

Polysomnographic & Other Objective Findings

Nocturnal polysomnography typically shows a prolonged total bed time with fragmented sleep. Sleep latency is prolonged, wake time after sleep onset is increased, and sleep efficiency is low. REM may be somewhat shortened in the case of untreated depression. Sleep latencies on the MSLT are often within normal limits, a result contrasting with the subjective complaint of severe daytime sleepiness. Twenty-four-hour continuous sleep recording studies typically show considerable time spent in bed during day and night. Psychiatric interviews and evaluations are essential to diagnose the underlying psychiatric condition.

Clinical & Pathologic Subtypes

Hypersomnia associated with a major depressive episode: Hypersomnia in the context of depression is a frequent feature of atypical depression and bipolar type II disorder (recurrent major depressive episodes with hypomanic episodes). MSLT results are normal, but long hours spent in bed are reported.

Hypersomnia as a conversion disorder or as an undifferentiated somatoform disorder: Pseudohypersomnia or pseudonarcolepsy, sometimes with pseudocataplexy, has been described.

Hypersomnia associated with seasonal affective disorder: Daytime fatigue, loss of concentration, increased appetite for carbohydrates, and weight gain are reported.

Differential Diagnosis

- Hypersomnia can occur in *idiopathic hypersomnia, narcolepsy, SRBDs, PLMD, behaviorally induced insufficient sleep syndrome,* and *environmental sleep disorder.*
- *Chronic fatigue syndrome* is characterized by persistent or relapsing fatigue that does not resolve with sleep or rest.

Physiological (Organic) Hypersomnia, Unspecified (Organic Hypersomnia, NOS) 327.10

Disorders that satisfy clinical criteria (a complaint of excessive sleepiness occurring almost daily for at least three months) and MSLT criteria (mean sleep latency less than eight minutes with fewer than two SOREMPs) for hypersomnolence and are believed to be due to a physiological condition, but do not meet criteria for other hypersomnolence conditions, are classified here.

IV. Circadian Rhythm Sleep Disorders

General Criteria for Circadian Rhythm Sleep Disorder

A. There is a persistent or recurrent pattern of sleep disturbance due primarily to one of the following:
  i. Alterations of the circadian timekeeping system
  ii. Misalignment between the endogenous circadian rhythm and exogenous factors that affect the timing or duration of sleep
B. The circadian related sleep disruption leads to insomnia, excessive daytime sleepiness, or both.
C. The sleep disturbance is associated with impairment of social, occupational, or other areas of functioning.

All disorders described in the ensuing sections imply a sleep difficulty that meets each of the above criteria. The specific features that characterize each type of circadian rhythm sleep disorder are included within the individual diagnostic criteria.

Diagnostic Criteria for

Circadian Rhythm Sleep Disorder, Delayed Sleep Phase Type (Delayed Sleep Phase Disorder) 327.31

A. There is a delay in the phase of the major sleep period in relation to the desired sleep time and wake-up time, as evidenced by a chronic or recurrent complaint of inability to fall asleep at a desired conventional clock time together with the inability to awaken at a desired and socially acceptable time.
B. When allowed to choose their preferred schedule, patients will exhibit normal sleep quality and duration for age and maintain a delayed, but stable, phase of entrainment to the 24-hour sleep-wake pattern.
C. Sleep log or actigraphy monitoring (including sleep diary) for at least seven days demonstrates a stable delay in the timing of the habitual sleep period.
Note: In addition, a delay in the timing of other circadian rhythms, such as the nadir of the core body temperature rhythm or DLMO, is useful for confirmation of the delayed phase.
D. The disturbance is not better explained by another sleep disorder, medical or neurological disorder, mental disorder, medication use, or substance use disorder.

Essential Features

Circadian rhythm sleep disorder, delayed sleep phase type (DSP) is characterized by habitual sleep-wake times that are delayed, usually more than two hours, relative to conventional or socially acceptable times. Affected individuals complain of difficulty falling asleep at a socially acceptable time, but once sleep ensues, sleep is reported to be normal. A typical patient has difficulty initiating sleep and prefers late wake-up times. Attempts to fall asleep earlier are usually unsuccessful.

Polysomnographic & Other Objective Findings

Recordings of sleep logs and actigraphy over a period of at least two weeks demonstrate delayed sleep onset and sleep offset. Sleep onset is typically delayed until 1 a.m. to 6 a.m., and wake time occurs in the late morning or afternoon. Daily demands and schedules may result in an earlier than desired wake-up time during weekdays, but a delay in bedtime and wake-up time is almost always seen during weekends and vacation.

Polysomnography, when performed at preferred (delayed) sleep times, is essentially normal for age. If a conventional bedtime and wake-up time is enforced, however, polysomnographic recording will show prolonged sleep latency and decreased total sleep time.

Laboratory measures of circadian timing generally show the expected phase delay in the timing of the nadir of the temperature rhythm and dim-light melatonin onset (DLMO). However, wake-up time may be even more delayed relative to these circadian markers.

The Horne-Östberg questionnaire is a useful tool to assess the chronotype of "eveningness" and "morningness." Individuals with circadian rhythm sleep disorder, delayed sleep phase type, score as definite evening types.

Differential Diagnosis

- Circadian rhythm sleep disorder, delayed sleep phase type, must be distinguished from "*normal*" sleep patterns, particularly in adolescents and young adults who maintain delayed schedules without distress or impaired functioning. Social and behavioral factors play an important role in the development and maintenance of the delayed sleep patterns. Personal, social, and occupational activities that continue into the late evening may perpetuate and exacerbate the sleep phase delay. In adolescents, the role of school avoidance, social maladjustment, and family dysfunction should be considered as contributing factors.

- Delayed sleep phase disorder must be distinguished from other causes of difficulty maintaining sleep, including *primary and secondary insomnias*. In DSP sleep initiation and maintenance are normal when the patient is allowed to sleep on the preferred schedule.
- The development of delayed sleep phase disorder is influenced by alterations in circadian physiology as well as behavioral factors. The *ICD-9-CM* includes a "behavioral" code for delayed sleep phase disorder. Although social, psychological, and environmental factors may play a significant role in the development of delayed sleep phase, *ICSD-2* has chosen to list only a single delayed sleep phase diagnosis, with the recognition that most cases reflect variable chronobiologic and behavioral contributions.

Diagnostic Criteria for

Circadian Rhythm Sleep Disorder, Advanced Sleep Phase Type (Advanced Sleep Phase Disorder) 327.32

A. There is an advance in the phase of the major sleep period in relation to the desired sleep time and wake-up time, as evidenced by a chronic or recurrent complaint of inability to stay awake until the desired conventional clock time, together with an inability to remain asleep until the desired and socially acceptable time for awakening.

B. When patients are allowed to choose their preferred schedule, sleep quality and duration are normal for age with an advanced, but stable, phase of entrainment to the 24-hour sleep-wake pattern.

C. Sleep logs or actigraphy monitoring (including sleep diaries) for at least seven days demonstrate a stable advance in the timing of the habitual sleep period.

Note: *In addition, an advance in the timing of other circadian rhythms such as the nadir of the core body temperature rhythm or DLMO, is useful for confirmation of the advanced circadian phase.*

D. The disturbance is not better explained by another sleep disorder, medical or neurological disorder, mental disorder, medication use, or substance use disorder.

Essential Features

Advanced sleep phase type (ASP), is a stable advance of the major sleep period characterized by habitual sleep onset and wake-up times that are several hours earlier relative to conventional and desired times. Affected individuals complain of sleepiness in the late afternoon or early evening, early sleep onset, and spontaneous early morning awakening. Individuals typically complain of early morning insomnia and excessive evening sleepiness. When patients are allowed to maintain an advanced schedule, their sleep is usually normal for age.

Polysomnographic & Other Objective Findings

Recording of sleep diary and actigraphy over a period of at least seven days demonstrates sleep onset and sleep offset that are advanced relative to conventional times. Sleep onset is typically advanced to between 6 p.m. and 9 p.m., and wake times to between 2 a.m. and 5 a.m. Daily demands may result in later than desired bedtimes. Polysomnography, when performed at the preferred sleep times (advanced), is essentially normal for age. However, if conventional bedtime and wake times are enforced, the polysomnographic recording may show decreased sleep latency, decreased total sleep time, and moderately short rapid eye movement sleep latency.

Laboratory measures to determine the phase of circadian rhythms generally show the expected phase advance in the timing of the nadir of the temperature rhythm and DLMO. However, wake-up time may be more advanced relative to these circadian markers. The Horne-Östberg questionnaire is a useful tool to assess the chronotype of "eveningness" and "morningness." Individuals with circadian rhythm sleep disorder, advanced sleep phase type, score as definite morning types.

Differential Diagnosis

- Advanced sleep phase type must be distinguished from "*normal*" sleep patterns, particularly in the elderly who maintain advanced schedules without distress or impaired functioning (morning types or larks).
- Advanced sleep phase disorder must be distinguished from other causes of early awakening, including *primary and secondary insomnia* problems.
- *Major depressive disorder* is a common cause of early awakening that must be considered. These patients do not typically manifest the early evening sleepiness that is characteristic of advanced sleep phase.

Diagnostic Criteria for

Circadian Rhythm Sleep Disorder, Irregular Sleep-Wake Type (Irregular Sleep-Wake Rhythm) 327.33

A. There is a chronic complaint of insomnia, excessive sleepiness, or both.

B. Sleep logs or actigraphy monitoring (including sleep diaries) for at least seven days demonstrate multiple irregular sleep bouts (at least three) during a 24-hour period.

C. Total sleep time per 24-hour period is essentially normal for age.

D. The disturbance is not better explained by another sleep disorder, medical or neurological disorder, mental disorder, medication use, or substance use disorder.

Essential Features

Circadian rhythm sleep disorder, irregular sleep-wake type, is characterized by lack of a clearly defined circadian rhythm of sleep and wake. The sleep-wake pattern is temporally disorganized so that sleep and wake periods are variable throughout the 24-hour period. Individuals have symptoms of insomnia and excessive sleepiness, depending on the time of day.

Polysomnographic & Other Objective Findings

Sleep logs and actigraphy monitoring show the expected lack of a clear circadian rhythm of the sleep-wake cycle which, instead, is characterized by multiple irregular sleep and wake bouts throughout the 24-hour period. Monitoring of other circadian rhythms, such as core body temperature, may also show a loss of circadian rhythmicity.

Differential Diagnosis

- *Poor sleep hygiene* and voluntary maintenance of irregular sleep schedules should be distinguished from irregular sleep-wake pattern.

- Irregular sleep and wake patterns associated with known neurological and medical conditions should be coded under *circadian rhythm sleep disorders due to medical condition*.

Diagnostic Criteria for

Circadian Rhythm Sleep Disorder, Free-Running Type (Nonentrained Type) 327.34

A. There is a complaint of insomnia or excessive sleepiness related to abnormal synchronization between the 24-hour light-dark cycle and the endogenous circadian rhythm of sleep and wake propensity.

B. Sleep log or actigraphy monitoring (with sleep diaries) for at least seven days demonstrates a pattern of sleep and wake times that typically delays each day with a period longer than 24 hours.

Note: *Monitoring sleep logs or actigraphy for more than seven days is preferred in order to clearly establish the daily drift.*

C. The disturbance is not better explained by another sleep disorder, medical or neurological disorder, mental disorder, medication use, or substance use disorder.

Essential Features

Circadian rhythm sleep disorder, free-running type, (nonentrained type) is characterized by sleep symptoms that occur because the intrinsic circadian pacemaker is not entrained to a 24-hour period or is free running with a non–24-hour period (usually slightly longer). Some individuals adopt a sleep pattern that is congruent with their free-running pacemaker and shift their sleep times each day in concert with their circadian rhythms.

Polysomnographic & Other Objective Findings

Recording of sleep logs and actigraphy over prolonged periods may demonstrate the lack of a stable relationship between the sleep-wake cycle and the 24-hour day. When sleep schedules follow the endogenous circadian propensity for sleep and wake, actigraphy and polysomnography are usually normal for age, but sleep-onset and wake times are typically delayed each day.

Serial measurements of circadian rhythms, such as the DLMO or the core body temperature rhythm, usually show a progressive daily delay of the phase of the rhythm consistent with a period that is longer than 24 hours.

Differential Diagnosis

- Some individuals with *circadian rhythm sleep disorder, delayed sleep phase type*, may demonstrate progressive delay of their sleep period for several days, and their symptoms may be confused with those of circadian rhythm sleep disorder, free-running type (nonentrained type).

- Behavioral factors and *psychiatric disorders*, as well as *medical and neurological disorders* (including, in particular, *blindness*, but also *dementia* or *mental retardation*), may play a role in the development of circadian rhythm disorder, free-running type. However, in many of these cases, multiple physiologic, behavioral and environmental factors contribute to the condition. In the majority of these cases, the disorder should be coded as circadian rhythm sleep disorder, free-running type. This includes free-running rhythms that are associated with blindness.

- If the sleep disorder is believed to be predominantly or exclusively socially or environmentally induced, then it should be coded as *other circadian rhythm sleep disorder (circadian rhythm sleep disorder, NOS)*. If there is evidence that the sleep disorder is predominantly or exclusively a function of medical or neurological disorders, then state and code as *circadian rhythm sleep disorder due to medical condition*.

Diagnostic Criteria for

Circadian Rhythm Sleep Disorder, Jet Lag Type (Jet Lag Disorder) 327.35

A. There is a complaint of insomnia or excessive daytime sleepiness associated with transmeridian jet travel across at least two time zones.

B. There is associated impairment of daytime function, general malaise, or somatic symptoms such as gastrointestinal disturbance within one to two days after travel.

C. The disturbance is not better explained by another sleep disorder, medical or neurological disorder, mental disorder, medication use, or substance use disorder.

Essential Features

Circadian rhythm sleep disorder, jet lag type, is a circadian rhythm sleep disorder in which there is a temporary mismatch between the timing of the sleep and wake cycle generated by the endogenous circadian clock and that of the sleep and wake pattern required by a change in time zone. Individuals complain of disturbed sleep, decreased subjective alertness, and impaired daytime function. The severity of symptoms is dependent on the number of time zones traveled and the direction of the travel. Eastward travel (requiring advancing circadian rhythms and sleep-wake hours) is usually more difficult to adjust to than westward travel.

Polysomnographic & Other Objective Findings

Objective laboratory testing is usually not indicated. When performed, polysomnography or actigraphy shows a loss of a normal sleep-wake pattern or a mismatch between the timing of sleep and wakefulness with the desired sleep-wake pattern of the local time.

Differential Diagnosis

- A thorough history and physical examination should be performed to exclude other mental, physical, or sleep disorders. Somatic complaints of gastrointestinal or urinary symptoms (*nocturia*) may indicate an underlying medical condition.
- When jet-lag symptoms persist, increasing frustration, negative expectations, and poor sleep hygiene may predispose the individual to the development of *psychophysiological insomnia*.

Diagnostic Criteria for

Circadian Rhythm Sleep Disorder, Shift Work Type (Shift Work Disorder) 327.36

A. There is a complaint of insomnia or excessive sleepiness that is temporally associated with a recurring work schedule that overlaps the usual time for sleep.
B. The symptoms are associated with the shift-work schedule over the course of at least one month.
C. Sleep log or actigraphy monitoring (with sleep diaries) for at least seven days demonstrates disturbed circadian and sleep-time misalignment.
D. The sleep disturbance is not better explained by another current sleep disorder, medical or neurological disorder, mental disorder, medication use, or substance use disorder.

Essential Features

Circadian rhythm sleep disorder, shift work type, is characterized by complaints of insomnia or excessive sleepiness that occur in relation to work hours that are scheduled during the usual sleep period. There are several types of shift-work schedules, including night shifts, early morning shifts, and rotating shifts. The sleep disturbance is most commonly reported in association with the night and early morning shifts. Total sleep time is typically curtailed by one to four hours in night and early morning shift workers, and sleep quality is perceived as unsatisfactory. In addition to impairment of performance at work, reduced alertness may also be associated with consequences for safety. The sleep disorder occurs despite attempts to optimize environmental conditions for sleep. The condition usually persists for the duration of the work-shift period. However, in some individuals, the sleep disturbance may persist beyond the duration of shift work.

Polysomnographic & Other Objective Findings

The condition can usually be diagnosed by history. Polysomnographic recordings may be useful if the sleep disorder is severe or the etiology of the sleep disturbance is in question. Ideally, the sleep recording is performed during the habitual "shifted" sleep period. Monitoring of an episode of usual daytime wakefulness and night sleep during a daytime shift is ideal for comparative purposes. Polysomnography may demonstrate impaired quality of the habitual sleep period, with either a prolonged sleep latency or shortened total sleep time, depending on the timing of the sleep period in relation to the underlying phase of the circadian timing system. The sleep period may be fragmented, with frequent arousals and awakenings. The MSLT may demonstrate excessive sleepiness during the time of the work shift.

Sleep diaries and actigraphy are very useful in demonstrating a disrupted sleep-wake pattern consistent with shift work sleep disorder. If available, measures of the unmasked melatonin or 24-hour temperature rhythm are useful to indicate the degree of circadian desynchrony.

Differential Diagnosis

- The excessive sleepiness should be differentiated from that due to other primary sleep disorders such as *OSA* or *narcolepsy*.
- *Insufficient sleep* related to conflicting daytime activities (e.g., child care) or from environmental interference with sleep (e.g., daytime noise) often contributes to sleepiness.
- Sometimes patients with *delayed sleep phase disorder* may adopt a night-work schedule that is more congruent with their sleep preferences.
- *Insomnia* and *excessive sleepiness* may suggest other persistent circadian rhythm sleep disorders. However, historical information on the relation between the occurrence of disturbed sleep and work-hour distribution should provide sufficient information to indicate the correct diagnosis.
- Increasing frustration, negative expectations, and poor sleep hygiene may predispose the person to the development of coexisting *psychophysiological insomnia.*
- *Drug and alcohol abuse or dependency* may result from efforts to treat the sleep disturbance.

Diagnostic Criteria for

Circadian Rhythm Sleep Disorder Due to Medical Condition 327.37

A. There is a complaint of insomnia or excessive sleepiness related to alterations of the circadian timekeeping system or a misalignment between the endogenous circadian rhythm and exogenous factors that affect the timing or duration of sleep.

B. An underlying medical or neurological disorder predominantly accounts for the circadian rhythm sleep disorder.

C. Sleep log or actigraphy monitoring (with sleep diaries) for at least seven days demonstrates disturbed or low amplitude circadian rhythmicity.

D. The sleep disturbance is not better explained by another current sleep disorder, mental disorder, medication use, or substance use disorder.

Essential Features

The etiology of the circadian rhythm sleep disorder is an underlying primary medical or neurological condition. Depending on the underlying neurological or medical disorder, patients may present with a variety of symptoms, including insomnia and excessive sleepiness. The sleep-wake pattern may range from alterations in phase to irregular sleep-wake patterns.

Polysomnographic & Other Objective Findings

Sleep studies yield different results depending on when they are performed and the alterations in sleep architecture that may accompany the underlying medical or neurological disorder. Recordings of sleep diaries and actigraphy over a period of at least two weeks demonstrate sleep onsets and sleep offsets that may be delayed or advanced relative to conventional times, irregular or free running. Laboratory measures to determine the phase and amplitude of circadian rhythms generally show the expected phase advance or delay of circadian rhythms or a decrease in the amplitude.

Differential Diagnosis

- The main difficulty in establishing the diagnosis is to determine whether the primary cause is a medical or neurological disorder or an alteration in exposure to circadian synchronizing agents such as light and activity.
- Depending upon the particular type of circadian disturbance, clinical presentations may suggest difficulty initiating or maintaining sleep or excessive sleepiness. See *Differential Diagnosis* sections for other specific circadian rhythm sleep disorders for additional discussion.

Other Circadian Rhythm Sleep Disorder (Circadian Rhythm Disorder, NOS) 327.39

Disorders that: 1) satisfy the criteria of a circadian rhythm sleep disorder, as defined above; 2) are not due to drug or substance; and 3) do not meet criteria for other circadian rhythm sleep disorders are classified here.

Other Circadian Rhythm Sleep Disorder Due to Drug or Substance 292.85 (for Alcohol use 291.82)

Disorders that: 1) satisfy the general criteria of a circadian rhythm sleep disorder, as defined above; 2) are due to a drug or substance; and 3) do not meet criteria for other circadian rhythm sleep disorders are classified here.

V. PARASOMNIAS

Parasomnias are undesirable physical events or experiences that occur during entry into sleep, within sleep, or during arousals from sleep. Parasomnias encompass abnormal sleep related movements, behaviors, emotions, perceptions, dreaming, and autonomic nervous system functioning. Parasomnias are clinical disorders because of the resulting injuries, sleep disruption, adverse health effects, and untoward psychosocial effects. Parasomnias can affect the patient, the bed partner, or both.

Abnormal sleep related movements comprise a subset of parasomnias that is detailed in the "Sleep Related Movement Disorders" section.

Parasomnias often involve complex, seemingly purposeful, and goal-directed behaviors, which presumably are performed with some personal meaning to the individual at the time, despite the illogical and unsound nature of the behaviors enacted outside the conscious awareness of the individual. Only one parasomnia in the *ICSD-2*, viz. RBD, requires polysomnographic documentation as one of the essential diagnostic criteria.

DISORDERS OF AROUSAL (FROM NON-RAPID EYE MOVEMENT SLEEP)

Diagnostic Criteria for

Confusional Arousals 327.41

A. Recurrent mental confusion or confusional behavior occurs during an arousal or awakening from nocturnal sleep or a daytime nap.
B. The disturbance is not better explained by another sleep disorder, medical or neurological disorder, mental disorder, medication use, or substance use disorder.

Alternate Names
Sleep drunkenness, (excessive) sleep inertia.

Essential Features

Confusional arousals consist of mental confusion or confusional behavior during or following arousals from sleep, typically from slow-wave sleep in the first part of the night, but also upon attempted awakening from sleep in the morning.

Associated Features

Sleep talking or occasional shouting is common during confusional arousals, and bruxism can also occur.

Familial Pattern

As in all of the disorders of arousal, genetic factors appear to play an important role.

Polysomnographic & Other Objective Findings

Confusional arousals typically arise from slow-wave sleep. They most often occur in the first third of the night but can also occur later in the night and from other NREM sleep stages and can even occur during daytime naps. Time-synchronized video recording is essential if polysomnography is to be used as support for the diagnosis. A normal polysomnogram does not rule out the diagnosis of confusional arousals.

Clinical or Pathologic Subtypes

In adolescents and adults, confusional arousals can have two variants: severe morning sleep inertia and sleep-related abnormal sexual behaviors. *Severe morning sleep inertia* occurs during the morning transition from sleep to wakefulness and appears to arise mainly from light NREM sleep. *Sleep related abnormal sexual behaviors* can primarily be classified as confusional arousals and include prolonged or violent masturbation, sexual molestation and assaults, initiation of sexual intercourse, and loud (sexual) vocalizations during sleep—followed by morning amnesia.

Differential Diagnosis

- Confusional arousals associated with *OSA* must be identified.
- *Nocturnal partial seizures* and medical disorders that could trigger or mimic confusional arousals should also be identified.
- *Sleepwalking* and *sleep terrors* can usually be distinguished from confusional arousals in childhood. However, there can be considerable

overlap among the three disorders of arousal, and also with *RBD*, in adults.

- Confusional arousals that are determined to be predominantly or exclusively induced by a drug, substance or medical condition in a given patient should be classified in the *"Parasomnia due to…"* sections of *ICSD-2*. In contrast, confusional arousals precipitated by a drug, substance or medical condition in a minority of episodes for a given patient should be classified as primary confusional arousals, as described in this section.

Diagnostic Criteria for

Sleepwalking 307.46

A. Ambulation occurs during sleep.
B. Persistence of sleep, an altered state of consciousness, or impaired judgment during ambulation is demonstrated by at least one of the following:
  i. Difficulty in arousing the person
  ii. Mental confusion when awakened from an episode
  iii. Amnesia (complete or partial) for the episode
  iv. Routine behaviors that occur at inappropriate times
  v. Inappropriate or nonsensical behaviors
  vi. Dangerous or potentially dangerous behaviors
C. The disturbance is not better explained by another sleep disorder, medical or neurological disorder, mental disorder, medication use, or substance use disorder.

Alternate Names
Somnambulism.

Essential Features
Sleepwalking consists of a series of complex behaviors that are usually initiated during arousals from slow-wave sleep and culminate in walking around with an altered state of consciousness and impaired judgment. Episodes often begin with sitting up in bed and looking about in a confused manner before walking; episodes can also begin with immediately leaving the bed and walking or even "bolting" from the bed and running. Frantic attempts to escape an imminent perceived or dreamed threat can occur. Agitated, belligerent, or violent behavior can also occur. There is usually

amnesia for these episodes, although adults can remember fragments of episodes and sometimes will have considerable recall for the events. Dreaming during sleepwalking is sometimes reported in adults. Sleep talking and shouting can accompany these events. The eyes are usually open during an episode and, not uncommonly, are wide open with a confused "glassy" stare, in contrast to RBD, when the eyes are usually closed during an episode. An episode of sleepwalking can occasionally occur during a daytime nap.

Associated Features
Violence is not uncommon with adult sleepwalking, especially in men, and a person attempting to awaken a sleepwalker during an episode can be violently attacked. On rare occasions, driving a car (including long distances), inadvertent homicide (including filicide), and pseudosuicide can occur during sleepwalking. Sleepwalking with indecent exposure or other paraphilic activity and other abnormal sleep related sexual behaviors have been reported, as has somnambulistic eating.

Familial Pattern
A strong familial pattern has been reported.

Polysomnographic & Other Objective Findings
Sleepwalking typically begins after an arousal from slow-wave sleep and occasionally from stage 2 NREM sleep. Heart rate acceleration, increased muscle tone, and muscle twitching rarely occur before a slow-wave sleep arousal. Heart rate acceleration emerges abruptly with the arousals from slow-wave sleep. Time-synchronized video recording is essential if polysomnography is to be used as support for the diagnosis. A normal polysomnogram does not rule out the diagnosis of sleepwalking.

Differential Diagnosis
- It can be difficult to distinguish agitated sleepwalking in adults or children from *sleep terrors*, since both states can manifest with screaming, bolting from bed and running, and violence.
- *RBD* typically presents as dream-enacting behaviors during the second half of the night and usually affects middle-aged men but can also affect both sexes and virtually any age group. Since sleepwalking in adults can also present as dream-enacting behaviors that can emerge during any time of the night, polysomnography may be necessary to distinguish sleepwalking from RBD.

- *Parasomnia overlap disorder* should be diagnosed if sleepwalking (or sleep terrors) occurs with RBD in the same patient.
- Other sleep disorders, such as *OSA*, can precipitate disordered arousals with ambulation, so a careful history must be obtained in the search for other sleep disorders.
- *Sleep related epilepsy* can manifest with wandering behavior or with frenzied walking or running.
- In adults, a diagnosis of *malingering* should also be considered.
- If a neurological or medical disorder is identified as the precipitant of sleepwalking, then the sleepwalking should be diagnosed as *parasomnia due to medical condition*.

Diagnostic Criteria for

Sleep Terrors 307.46

A. A sudden episode of terror occurs during sleep, usually initiated by a cry or loud scream that is accompanied by autonomic nervous system and behavioral manifestations of intense fear.
B. At least one of the following associated features is present:
    i. Difficulty in arousing the person
    ii. Mental confusion when awakened from an episode
    iii. Amnesia (complete or partial) for the episode
    iv. Dangerous or potentially dangerous behaviors
C. The disturbance is not better explained by another sleep disorder, medical or neurological disorder, mental disorder, medication use, or substance use disorder.

Alternate Names
Night terrors, *pavor nocturnus*.

Essential Features
Sleep terrors consist of arousals from slow-wave sleep accompanied by a cry or piercing scream and autonomic nervous system and behavioral manifestations of intense fear. There is often intense autonomic discharge, with tachycardia, tachypnea, flushing of the skin, diaphoresis, mydriasis, and increased muscle tone. The person usually sits up in bed; is unresponsive to external stimuli; and, if awakened, is confused and disoriented. However, bolting

out of bed and running is not uncommon in adults and can also be associated with violent behaviors. Amnesia for the episode subsequently occurs, although sometimes there are reports of dream fragments or brief vivid dream images or hallucinations. In some adults, more elaborate dream imagery can be reported, especially in regard to a frightening encounter. The sleep terror episode may be accompanied by incoherent vocalizations.

Familial Pattern
Sleep terrors can occur in several members of a family.

Polysomnographic & Other Objective Findings
A sleep terror typically begins after a sudden arousal from slow-wave sleep, most commonly toward the end of the first or second episode of slow-wave sleep. The information on other objective findings described for sleepwalking also applies to sleep terrors. Time-synchronized video recording is essential if polysomnography is to be used as support for the diagnosis. A normal polysomnogram does not rule out the diagnosis of sleep terrors.

Differential Diagnosis
- Sleep terrors can be readily distinguished from *sleepwalking* and *confusional arousals* in children but not as easily in adults, who show considerable overlap among the disorders of arousal as well as between these disorders and *RBD*.
- *Parasomnia overlap disorder* should be diagnosed if sleep terrors (or sleepwalking) occur with RBD. If a neurological or medical disorder is identified as the precipitant of sleep terrors, then the sleep terrors should be diagnosed as *parasomnia due to medical condition*.
- Also, *nocturnal complex partial seizures, frontal lobe seizures,* and *nocturnal panic attacks* can mimic sleep terrors. Seizures typically involve repetitive stereotypic behaviors (with or without any associated epileptiform activity in the scalp EEG), and panic attacks usually occur during a full awakening with immediate awareness that a panic attack is taking place.
- In adults, a diagnosis of *malingering* should also be considered.

PARASOMNIAS USUALLY ASSOCIATED WITH RAPID EYE MOVEMENT SLEEP

Diagnostic Criteria for

> ### Rapid Eye Movement Sleep Behavior Disorder (Including Parasomnia Overlap Disorder and Status Dissociatus) 327.42
>
> A. Presence of REM sleep without atonia: the EMG finding of excessive amounts of sustained or intermittent elevation of submental EMG tone or excessive phasic submental or (upper or lower) limb EMG twitching.
>
> B. At least one of the following is present:
>
>   i. Sleep related injurious, potentially injurious, or disruptive behaviors by history
>
>   ii. Abnormal REM sleep behaviors documented during polysomnographic monitoring
>
>   iii. Awakening short of breath
>
> C. Absence of EEG epileptiform activity during REM sleep unless RBD can be clearly distinguished from any concurrent REM sleep-related seizure disorder.
>
> D. The sleep disturbance is not better explained by another sleep disorder, medical or neurological disorder, mental disorder, medication use, or substance use disorder.

Essential Features

REM sleep behavior disorder (RBD) is characterized by abnormal behaviors emerging during REM sleep that cause injury or sleep disruption. RBD is also associated with EMG abnormalities during REM sleep. The EMG demonstrates an excess of muscle tone or phasic EMG twitch activity during REM sleep. A complaint of sleep related injury is common with RBD, which usually manifests as an attempted enactment of distinctly altered, unpleasant, action-filled, and violent dreams in which the individual is being confronted, attacked, or chased by unfamiliar people or animals. Typically, at the end of an episode, the individual awakens quickly; becomes rapidly alert; and reports a dream with a coherent story, with the dream action corresponding to the observed sleep behaviors. Sleep and dream related behaviors reported by history and documented during polysomnography include talking, laughing, shouting, swearing, gesturing, reaching, grabbing, arm flailing, slapping, punching, kicking, sitting up, leaping from bed, crawling, and running.

Walking, however, is quite uncommon with RBD, and leaving the room is especially rare and probably accidental. The eyes usually remain closed during an RBD episode, with the person attending to the dream action and not to the actual environment; this is a major reason for the high rate of injury in RBD. Also, chewing, feeding, drinking, sexual behaviors, urination, and defecation have not been documented to occur in REM sleep, which mirrors the findings from an animal model of RBD. Because RBD occurs during REM sleep, it usually appears at least 90 minutes after sleep onset unless there is coexisting narcolepsy, in which case RBD can emerge shortly after sleep onset during a sleep-onset REM period. RBD is usually a longstanding and progressive disorder. There is an acute form of RBD that emerges during intense REM sleep rebound states, such as during withdrawal from alcohol and sedative-hypnotic agents, with certain medication use, or with drug intoxication.

Associated Features
PLMS is very common with RBD and may disturb the sleep of the bed partner. Daytime tiredness or sleepiness is uncommon unless narcolepsy is also present. There is typically no history of irritable, aggressive, or violent behavior during the day.

Demographics
RBD is a male-predominant disorder that usually emerges after the age of 50 years, although any age group can be affected. One third of patients with newly diagnosed Parkinson's disease have RBD, and 90% of patients with multiple system atrophy have RBD.

Predisposing & Precipitating Factors
An increasingly recognized precipitating factor is medication use, particularly venlafaxine, selective serotonin reuptake inhibitors, mirtazapine, and other antidepressant agents with the exception of buproprion.

Onset, Course, & Complications
Delayed emergence of a neurodegenerative disorder, often more than a decade after the onset of RBD, is very common in men 50 years of age and older. These disorders include Parkinson's disease, multiple system atrophy, Lewy body dementia, and others.

Polysomnographic & Other Objective Findings
There is an excessive amount of sustained EMG activity or intermittent loss of REM atonia or excessive phasic muscle twitch

activity of the submental or limb EMG during REM sleep, as documented by polysomnography. Autonomic nervous system activation (e.g., tachycardia) is uncommon during REM sleep motor activation in RBD, in contrast to the disorders of arousal. Approximately 75% of patients have PLMS during NREM sleep; a low percentage of these leg movements are associated with EEG signs of arousal. Increased percentages of slow-wave sleep and increased delta power in RBD have been found in controlled and uncontrolled studies. Sleep architecture, and the customary cycling among REM and NREM sleep stages, are usually preserved in RBD. Time-synchronized video recording is essential for helping establish the diagnosis of RBD during polysomnography.

Clinical or Pathophysiological Subtypes

Subclinical RBD consists of the REM sleep polysomnographic abnormalities of RBD but without a clinical history of RBD. There can be some minor subclinical REM sleep behaviors, such as limb twitching or jerking and talking, but no complex behaviors. *Parasomnia overlap disorder* consists of RBD combined with a disorder of arousal. Diagnostic criteria for both RBD and a disorder or disorders of arousal must be met. *Status dissociatus* can be classified as a subtype of RBD that manifests as an extreme form of state dissociation without identifiable sleep stages but with sleep and dream-related behaviors that closely resemble RBD. Status dissociatus represents a major breakdown of the polysomnographic markers for REM sleep, NREM sleep, and wakefulness, with admixtures of these states being present, but with conventional sleep stages not being identifiable during polysomnographic monitoring. There is abnormal behavioral release that can be associated with disturbed dreaming that closely resembles RBD.

Differential Diagnosis

- RBD is one of several disorders that can manifest as complex, injurious, and violent sleep-related and dream-related behaviors in adults, and it is one of various disorders that can disrupt the sleep of children. Other disorders that can mimic RBD in adults or children include *sleepwalking, sleep terrors, nocturnal seizures, OSA, hypnogenic paroxysmal dystonia, RMD, sleep related dissociative disorder, frightening hypnopompic hallucinations,* and *posttraumatic stress disorder;* a diagnosis of *malingering* should also be considered.

Diagnostic Criteria for

Recurrent Isolated Sleep Paralysis 327.43

A. The patient complains of an inability to move the trunk and all limbs at sleep onset or on waking from sleep.
B. Each episode lasts seconds to a few minutes.
C. The sleep disturbance is not better explained by another sleep disorder (particularly narcolepsy), a medical or neurological disorder, mental disorder, medication use, or substance use disorder.

Essential Features

Recurrent isolated sleep paralysis is characterized by an inability to perform voluntary movements at sleep onset (hypnagogic or predormital form) or on waking from sleep (hypnopompic or postdormital form) in the absence of a diagnosis of narcolepsy. The event is characterized by an inability to speak or to move the limbs, trunk, and head. Respiration is usually unaffected. Consciousness is preserved, and full recall is present.

Associated Features

Hallucinatory experiences may accompany the paralysis in about 25% to 75% of patients. These may include auditory, visual, or tactile hallucinations or the sense of a presence in the room.

Polysomnographic & Other Objective Findings

Studies of sleep paralysis arising after forced awakenings during the night have shown onset chiefly from REM sleep. During the episodes, the polysomnogram shows a dissociated state with either intrusion of alpha rhythm into REM sleep or persistence of REM-type atonia into wakefulness. The common feature is electromyographic atonia during the episode of paralysis.

Differential Diagnosis

- Sleep paralysis should be differentiated from transient compression *neuropathies*.
- *Cataplexy* produces similar generalized paralysis of skeletal muscles but occurs during wakefulness and is precipitated by emotion.
- *Atonic seizures* occur during wakefulness.

- *Nocturnal panic attacks* are not usually associated with paralysis.
- *Conversion disorders* may mimic sleep paralysis, but the clinical features are usually sufficiently different to make distinction easy.
- Familial periodic paralysis syndromes, especially *hypokalemic periodic paralysis*, may occur at rest and on awakening. However the episodes usually last hours, may be associated with carbohydrate intake, and are usually accompanied by hypokalemia. There are also hyperkalemic and normokalemic periodic paralysis syndromes.

Diagnostic Criteria for

Nightmare Disorder 307.47

A. Recurrent episodes of awakenings from sleep with recall of intensely disturbing dream mentation, usually involving fear or anxiety, but also anger, sadness, disgust, and other dysphoric emotions.

B. Full alertness on awakening, with little confusion or disorientation; recall of sleep mentation is immediate and clear.

C. At least one of the following associated features is present:
   i. Delayed return to sleep after the episodes
   ii. Occurrence of episodes in the latter half of the habitual sleep period

Alternate Names
Nightmares.

Essential Features
Nightmare disorder is characterized by recurrent nightmares, which are disturbing mental experiences that generally occur during REM sleep and that often result in awakening. Nightmares are coherent dream sequences that seem real and become increasingly more disturbing as they unfold. Emotions usually involve anxiety, fear, or terror but frequently also anger, rage, embarrassment, disgust, and other negative feelings. Dream content most often focuses on imminent physical danger to the individual but may also involve other distressing themes. Ability to detail the nightmare's contents upon awakening is common in nightmare disorder. Because nightmares typically arise during REM sleep, they may occur at any moment

that REM propensity is high. Nightmares arising either immediately following a trauma (ASD) or one month or more after a trauma (PTSD) can occur during NREM sleep, especially stage 2, as well as during REM sleep and at sleep onset.

Predisposing & Precipitating Factors

The clinical use of pharmacologic agents affecting the neurotransmitters norepinephrine, serotonin, and dopamine are associated with the complaint of nightmares. A majority of these agents are antidepressants, antihypertensives, and dopamine-receptor agonists. Agents affecting the neurotransmitters GABA, acetylcholine, and histamine, agents affecting the sleep related immunologic response to infectious disease, and the withdrawal of REM-sleep suppressive agents can also be associated with the complaint of nightmares.

Polysomnographic & Other Objective Findings

Polysomnographic recordings during actual nightmares are few in number and, in some instances, have shown abrupt awakenings from REM sleep preceded by accelerated heart and respiratory rates.

Differential Diagnosis

- Rare cases of *seizures* presenting as "nightmares" have been reported.
- Nightmares differ from *sleep terrors* in having detailed recollection of dreaming in contrast to fragments of dreams or no dream recall, presenting no or minimal overt movement or autonomic activity, occurring late in the night, being followed by rapid awakening and a difficult return to sleep, and often involving REM sleep.
- *RBD* occurs more often in late middle-aged men and is more often associated with violent explosive movements and a history of nocturnal injuries. The dream disturbance usually involves being threatened or attacked by unfamiliar people or animals and is controlled in tandem with the sleep behavioral disturbance by appropriate medication.
- Anxiety may accompany episodes of *sleep paralysis* occurring either at sleep onset (hypnagogic) or offset (hypnopompic), when the individual feels

conscious but unable to move, speak, and, at times, breathe properly.

- Patients with *narcolepsy* often report nightmares; these may occur at sleep onset. However, narcolepsy and nightmare disorder are clearly distinguishable by other clinical symptoms.

- *Nocturnal panic attacks* occur either during or immediately after nocturnal awakenings from NREM sleep.

- *Sleep related dissociative disorders* comprise a sleep related variant of the dissociative disorders as defined by the *DSM-IV,* including dissociative identity disorder (formerly called multiple personality disorder) and dissociative fugue, in which individuals meeting waking criteria for these diagnoses may at times experience the recall of actual physical or emotional trauma as a "dream" during periods of EEG-documented nocturnal waking.

- Nightmares that occur intermittently during the course of *ASD* or *PTSD* are an expected symptom of those mental disorders and do not require independent coding as nightmare disorder. However, when the frequency and/or severity of post-traumatic nightmares are such that they require independent clinical attention, then a diagnosis of nightmare disorder should be applied. In some cases, other symptoms of PTSD may have largely resolved while the nightmares persist. Nightmare disorder should be coded in these cases as well.

OTHER PARASOMNIAS

Diagnostic Criteria for

Sleep Related Dissociative Disorders 300.15

A. A dissociative disorder, fulfilling Diagnostic and Statistical Manual of Mental Disorders, Fourth Edition diagnostic criteria is present and emerges in close association with the main sleep period.

B. One of the following is present:
   i. Polysomnography demonstrates a dissociative episode or episodes that emerge during sustained EEG wakefulness, either in the transition from wakefulness to sleep or after an awakening from NREM or REM sleep
   ii. In the absence of a polysomnographically-recorded episode of dissociation, the history provided by observers is compelling for a sleep related dissociative disorder, particularly if the sleep related behaviors are similar to observed daytime dissociative behaviors

C. The sleep disturbance is not better explained by another sleep disorder, medical or neurologic disorder, medication use, or substance use disorder.

Alternate Names
Nocturnal (psychogenic) dissociative disorders.

Essential Features
Sleep related dissociative disorders are dissociative disorders that can emerge throughout the sleep period during well-established EEG wakefulness, either at the transition from wakefulness to sleep or within several minutes after an awakening from stages 1 or 2 NREM sleep or from REM sleep. Sleep related dissociative disorders comprise a sleep-related variant of dissociative disorders, which are defined in the *DSM-IV* as "…a disruption in the usually integrated functions of consciousness, memory, identity, or perception of the environment."

Associated Features
Most patients with sleep related dissociative disorders also have corresponding daytime dissociative disorders and have past or current histories of physical or sexual abuse. The episodes, which can be elaborate and last several minutes to an hour or longer,

often involve behaviors that represent reenactments of previous physical and sexual abuse situations. This activity may occur with perceived dreaming, which is actually a dissociated wakeful memory of past abuse. Sexualized behavior can occur and can be paired with defensive behavior and with congruent verbalization. Other dissociative episodes may occur as confusional states, with or without elaborate behaviors, which are not associated with perceived dreaming. The individual is usually completely amnestic for the behaviors expressed during a nocturnal dissociative episode.

Demographics
Sleep related dissociative disorders are predominant in females.

Predisposing & Precipitating Factors
A past or current history of physical, sexual, or verbal-emotional abuse, along with a severe and chronic history of psychiatric disorders, is the major predisposing and precipitating factor.

Polysomnographic & Other Objective Findings
In polysomnographic recordings of sleep related dissociative episodes, EEG wakefulness has been present before, during, and after the episodes. With disorders of arousal, the behaviors emerge almost immediately after the EEG arousal. With sleep related dissociative disorders, there is often a lag time of 15 to 60 seconds between EEG arousal and behavioral activation. Finally, polysomnographic monitoring may not capture a dissociative episode but is valuable in helping exclude other diagnostic possibilities.

Differential Diagnosis
- S*leepwalking, sleep terrors,* and *RBD* can share some overlapping features with sleep related dissociative disorders, but they usually have a shorter duration and the observed behaviors often can be distinguished from dissociative behaviors.
- Abnormal *toxic-metabolic states* or *medical disorders* that can cause altered states of consciousness may mimic a dissociative disorder and must be excluded.

Sleep Enuresis
Please see the Pediatric section of the Manual for this diagnosis.

Diagnostic Criteria for

Sleep Related Groaning (Catathrenia) 327.49

A *or* B satisfies the criteria:

A. A history of regularly occurring groaning (or related monotonous vocalization) occurring during sleep.

B. Polysomnography with respiratory-sound monitoring reveals a characteristic respiratory dysrhythmia predominantly or exclusively during REM sleep.

Alternate Names

Nocturnal groaning.

Essential Features

Sleep related groaning is a chronic, usually nightly, disorder characterized by expiratory groaning during sleep, particularly during the second half of the night. The groaning is not associated with any observed respiratory distress or anguished or emotional facial expression even though moaning and "mournful sounds" can occur. These recurrent bradypneic episodes may closely resemble central sleep apneas, although there are usually distinguishable differences between the two conditions.

Associated Features

The affected person is usually unaware of the groaning, and it is the bed partner, roommate, or family member or members who are disturbed by it and urge clinical evaluation. The groaning is usually loud and is not associated with any abnormal motor activity, sleep talking, or dreaming. However, the groaning usually stops whenever the person changes position in bed, only to resume again later. General physical examinations and routine laboratory testing, along with neurologic and otorhinolaryngologic examinations, are unremarkable. The affected person usually has no sleep related complaint. Hoarseness in the morning has also been reported. No association with respiratory disorders or with psychological problems or psychiatric disorders has been found.

Polysomnographic & Other Objective Findings

A characteristic respiratory dysrhythmia with inter-groaning intervals during sleep has been detected in all reported patients. Monitoring respiratory sound signals during sleep is required for identifying vocalizations. Groaning and moaning sounds usually start two to six hours after sleep onset, last 2 to 49 seconds, often repeat in clusters for two minutes to one hour, and may recur many times per night, predominantly or exclusively during REM sleep. The vocal sounds occur only during expiration. During the groaning, the person remains still. The sleep architecture is generally normal.

Differential Diagnosis

- *CSA* may be confused with the bradypneic events, but the presence of vocalizations indicates ongoing breathing rather than the cessation of breathing.
- *Sleep talking* involves the production of words and speech. Moaning can also occur during epileptic seizures.
- *Snoring* is an inspiratory noise caused by vibrations of the soft parts of the oropharyngeal walls.
- *Stridor* can be either inspiratory or expiratory and may occur exclusively during sleep. Unlike sleep related groaning, stridor may occur with every breath and not in clusters and tends not to occur as a prolonged expiration. In multiple system atrophy, however, stridor may occur in prolonged clusters (especially in REM sleep) that are interspersed with quiet breathing, but the stridor is always inspiratory.
- *Sleep related laryngospasm* usually is accompanied by a sense of suffocation.
- *Nocturnal asthma* with bronchoconstriction is accompanied by wheezing.

Diagnostic Criteria for

Exploding Head Syndrome 327.49

A. The patient complains of a sudden loud noise or sense of explosion in the head either at the wake-sleep transition or upon waking during the night.

B. The experience is not associated with significant pain complaints.

C. The patient rouses immediately after the event, usually with a sense of fright.

Note: In a minority of cases, a flash of light or myoclonic jerk may accompany the event.

Essential Features

Exploding head syndrome is characterized by a sudden, loud, imagined noise or sense of a violent explosion in the head occurring as the patient is falling asleep or waking during the night.

Polysomnographic & Other Objective Findings

Based on limited polysomnographic recordings, the events appear to arise from early drowsiness with predominant alpha rhythm, with interspersed theta activity. Slow eye movements have been noted. Arousals occur immediately following the episodes. No epileptiform activity has been reported. These findings are typical of a hypnagogic phenomenon.

Differential Diagnosis

- Exploding head syndrome should be distinguished from sudden-onset *headache syndromes*. In contrast to headache syndromes, exploding head syndrome is usually painless.
- *Simple partial seizures* can present with sensory phenomena but do not usually occur predominantly at sleep onset.
- *Nocturnal panic attacks* can awaken a person from sleep but are not usually associated with a sense of noise or explosion.
- Recurrent *nightmares* are characterized by recall of more complex and longer-lasting visual imagery.
- *Sleep starts* occur at the wake-sleep transition but are predominantly a motor phenomenon with sudden myoclonic jerks rather than an emphasis on sensory symptoms.

Diagnostic Criteria for

Sleep Related Hallucinations 368.16

A. The patient experiences hallucinations just prior to sleep onset or on awakening during the night or in the morning.

B. The hallucinations are predominantly visual.

Note: Hypnagogic or hypnopompic hallucinations may be difficult to differentiate from sleep-onset or sleep-termination dreaming. Complex nocturnal visual hallucinations may clearly occur in wakefulness following sudden arousal during the night.

C. The disturbance is not better explained by another sleep disorder, medical or neurological disorder, mental disorder, medication use, or substance use disorder.

Alternate Names

Hypnagogic hallucinations, hypnopompic hallucinations, complex nocturnal visual hallucinations.

Essential Features

Sleep related hallucinations are hallucinatory experiences, principally visual, that occur at sleep onset or on awakening from sleep. Hallucinations at sleep onset (hypnagogic hallucinations) may be difficult to differentiate from sleep-onset dreaming. Hallucinations on waking in the morning (hypnopompic hallucinations) may arise out of a period of REM sleep, and patients may also be uncertain whether they represent waking or dream-related experiences. Complex nocturnal visual hallucinations may represent a distinct form of sleep related hallucinations. They typically occur following a sudden awakening, without recall of a preceding dream. They usually take the form of complex, vivid, relatively immobile, images of people or animals, sometimes distorted in shape or size. These hallucinations may remain present for many minutes but usually disappear if ambient illumination is increased. Patients are clearly awake but often initially perceive the hallucinations as real and frightening.

Associated Features

Sleep related hallucinations may be associated with episodes of sleep paralysis, either at the same time or on different nights. Patients with complex nocturnal visual hallucinations may jump out of the bed in terror, sometimes injuring themselves. Some patients may experience other parasomnias, such as sleep talking or sleepwalking, separate from the hallucinations; some patients also may experience similar complex hallucinations during the day, unassociated with sleep.

Polysomnographic & Other Objective Findings

Sleep related hallucinations appear to arise predominantly from SOREMPs. However, the very few reports of polysomnography in complex nocturnal visual hallucinations suggest an onset out of NREM sleep. MRI scans of the brain, polysomnography, EEG and neuropsychometric testing may help in the differential diagnosis and in identifying underlying disorders.

Differential Diagnosis

- *Nightmares* are frightening dreams awakening the patient from sleep. They are clearly recognized as dreams and do not persist into wakefulness.
- *Exploding head syndrome* consists of a sudden sensation of an explosion in the head, usually at sleep onset and sometimes accompanied by a noise or flash of light. It does not involve complex visual imagery and lasts only seconds.

- In *RBD*, the patient acts out dreams during REM sleep. If not awakened by an observer, the person usually has little recollection of dream content.
- *Sleepwalking* may occasionally be associated with dream ideation, but the patient recognizes that the dream occurred during sleep.
- Visual hallucinations can be due to *epileptic seizures* but are usually brief, stereotyped, and fragmentary in such cases.
- Occasionally, complex visual hallucinations may be associated with *migraine* but are usually followed by a headache and rarely would wake a patient from sleep.
- Complex nocturnal visual hallucinations may be seen in patients with *narcolepsy, Parkinson's disease, dementia with Lewy bodies, visual loss (Charles Bonnet hallucinations),* and *midbrain and diencephalic pathology (peduncular hallucinosis),* as well as with the use of β-adrenergic receptor-blocking *medications.*
- *Anxiety disorders* have been noted in some patients.

Diagnostic Criteria for

Sleep Related Eating Disorder 327.49

A. Recurrent episodes of involuntary eating and drinking occur during the main sleep period.
B. One or more of the following must be present with the recurrent episodes of involuntary eating and drinking:
    i. Consumption of peculiar forms or combinations of food or inedible or toxic substances
    ii. Insomnia related to sleep disruption from repeated episodes of eating, with a complaint of nonrestorative sleep, daytime fatigue, or somnolence
    iii. Sleep-related injury
    iv. Dangerous behaviors performed while in pursuit of food or while cooking food
    v. Morning anorexia
    vi. Adverse health consequences from recurrent binge eating of high-caloric foods
C. The disturbance is not better explained by another sleep disorder, medical or neurological disorder, mental disorder, medication use, or substance use disorder.

Essential Features

Sleep related eating disorder (SRED) consists of recurrent episodes of involuntary eating and drinking during arousals from sleep with problematic consequences. The episodes of eating typically occur during partial arousals from sleep with subsequent partial recall. Some patients cannot be easily brought to full consciousness during an episode of eating. On the other hand, some patients seemingly have considerable alertness during an episode and have substantial recall in the morning.

Associated Features

Nightly frequency of eating, including multiple times nightly, is reported by a majority of affected individuals. The episodes of eating occur during any time in the sleep cycle. High-caloric foods are preferentially consumed.

Demographics

Females comprise 66% to 83% of patients in reported series. The mean age of onset of SRED is reported to be 22 to 29 years.

Predisposing & Precipitating Factors

SRED can be idiopathic, but it appears to be most commonly associated with a primary sleep disorder or other clinical condition. Sleepwalking is the most common sleep disorder associated with SRED; other sleep disorders include RLS, PLMD, OSA and circadian rhythm disorders. Medication-induced SRED has been reported with zolpidem, triazolam, and various other psychotropic agents. SRED can also be associated with daytime eating disorders and with a sleep related dissociative disorder.

Polysomnographic & Other Objective Findings

The most common findings are multiple confusional arousals, with or without eating, arising from slow-wave sleep. However, abnormal arousals have been documented from all stages of NREM sleep and also occasionally from REM sleep. PLMS and obstructive apneas may also be observed on polysomnography.

Differential Diagnosis

- Inappropriate compensatory behavior—such as self-induced vomiting; misuse of enemas, laxatives, diuretics or other medications; or other purging activity—should not be present in SRED; otherwise, the diagnosis of *bulimia nervosa* should be considered. However, a person with a daytime eating disorder can also have a coexisting SRED that is associated with confusional arousals but not associated with purging behaviors during the night or upon arising in the morning. Some patients with longstanding SRED and excessive weight gain may eventually fast during the daytime or engage in excessive exercise to prevent obesity as a result of the relentless SRED.

- Medical conditions that can cause recurrent eating in association with the main sleep period (besides during wakefulness) include *hypoglycemic states, peptic ulcer disease, reflux esophagitis, Kleine-Levin syndrome, Klüver-Bucy syndrome*, and others.

- SRED must primarily be distinguished from night eating syndrome (*NES*), which is characterized by the following features: overeating between the evening meal and nocturnal sleep onset, eating during complete awakenings from sleep with full subsequent recall, absence of bizarre (or toxic) food and substance ingestion and peculiar eating behaviors, and absence of an associated primary sleep disorder. SRED should also be distinguished from nocturnal (sleep related) extensions of *bulimia nervosa, binge-eating disorder,* and *anorexia nervosa, binge/purge type.*

- *Kleine-Levin syndrome* can present with inappropriate nocturnal eating, but its predominance in adolescent males and its hallmark symptom complex of periodic hypersomnia, hypersexuality, and hyperphagia lasting days to weeks should easily distinguish it from SRED. *Medical and neurological disorders* associated with abnormal recurrent eating should also be excluded.

VI. Sleep Related Movement Disorders

Sleep related movement disorders are conditions that are primarily characterized by relatively simple, usually stereotyped, movements that disturb sleep. RLS, although not involving stereotyped movements per se, is classified here mainly because of its close association with PLMD. The limb movements in RLS are complex and serve the purpose of avoiding the unpleasant sensations of that condition.

Nocturnal sleep disturbance or complaints of daytime sleepiness or fatigue are a prerequisite for a diagnosis of a sleep related movement disorder.

Body movements that disturb sleep are also seen in many other sleep disorder categories, e.g., in parasomnias such as sleepwalking, sleep terrors, and RBD. However, these parasomnias differ from the simple stereotyped movements in this category. In general, such parasomnias involve complex behaviors during the sleep period that may appear purposeful and goal-directed but are outside the conscious awareness of the individual.

There are some movement disorders that may occur during both sleep and wakefulness. If the presentation during sleep is significantly different from that during wakefulness, then the movement disorder is classified here. An example would be sleep related bruxism.

Some types of movements are typical of normal sleep, such as occasional sleep starts (hypnic jerks). However, in some patients, the frequency and intensity of these movements may be increased to the point where they severely disturb sleep. Setting a dividing line between normal and pathologic is very difficult in such cases.

Although the history may be telling, polysomnography may be necessary to make a firm diagnosis of sleep related movement disorders or parasomnias. Indeed, in some cases it may be necessary to add all-night videotaping to the usual polysomnographic recording and to correlate the documented movements with the technician's description of the patient's behavior and level of consciousness to establish a firm diagnosis.

Note: *Separate diagnostic criteria for RLS have been developed for young children who have difficulty reporting symptoms. The childhood criteria include the adult criteria and additional criteria designed to address the absence or uncertainty of verbal reports. See the Pediatric section of this Manual for the childhood criteria.*

Diagnostic Criteria for

Restless Legs Syndrome 333.99
Diagnosis in Adult Patients (Age Older Than 12 Years)

A. The patient reports an urge to move the legs, usually accompanied or caused by uncomfortable and unpleasant sensations in the legs.

B. The urge to move or the unpleasant sensations begin or worsen during periods of rest or inactivity such as lying or sitting

C. The urge to move or the unpleasant sensations are partially or totally relieved by movement, such as walking or stretching, at least as long as the activity continues.

D. The urge to move or the unpleasant sensations are worse, or only occur, in the evening or night.

E. The disorder is not better explained by another current sleep disorder, medical or neurological disorder, medication use, or substance use disorder.

Restless Legs Syndrome, Pediatric Diagnosis
Please see the Pediatric section of the Manual for more information.

Alternate Names
Ekbom's syndrome.

Essential Features
RLS is a sensorimotor disorder characterized by a complaint of a nearly irresistible urge to move the legs. This urge to move is often, but not always, accompanied by other uncomfortable paresthesias felt deep inside the legs. When paresthesias are present, the sensation may vary from uncomfortable to painful. The urge to move and any accompanying sensations are engendered or made worse by rest (lying or sitting) and are at least partially and temporarily relieved by walking or moving the legs. The relief is usually immediate. The urge to move the legs worsens in the evening or night with relative relief in the morning. The symptoms disturb quiet resting and often profoundly disturb the patient's ability to go to sleep or to return to sleep after an awakening. Patients may complain of involuntary jerking or twitching movements of the legs while sitting or lying awake. These may take the form of PLMW.

Associated Features
A motor expression of the disorder characterized as periodic

limb movements may occur in sleep (PLMS) and resting wakefulness (PLMW); these are most common in the legs, but the arms may be involved as well. PLMS occur in 80% to 90% of patients with RLS but are not specific for RLS.

Familial Patterns
More than 50% of patients with primary RLS report a familial pattern.

Polysomnographic & Other Objective Findings
PLMS occur in 80% to 90% of patients with RLS when the study is limited to one night.

Clinical & Pathophysiological Subtypes
Secondary RLS, caused by another disorder or condition, has been clearly shown to exist in pregnancy, end-stage renal disease, and iron deficiency. Primary RLS has two phenotypes: the early-onset phenotype of RLS tends to have an earlier age of onset, a more gradually progressive natural course, and a more common occurrence of RLS among family members compared to the late-onset phenotype.

Differential Diagnosis
- *Positional discomfort*, sometimes confused with RLS, can occur from pressure that compresses nerves, limits blood flow, or stretches body tissue. The discomfort is resolved by changing body position without requiring any continued movement. The discomfort does not include an urge to move the legs.
- *Sleep starts (hypnic jerks)* produce leg movements during the transition from sleep to waking, but the movements are involuntary with no urge to move the legs.
- *Neuroleptic-induced akathisia* differs from RLS in the generalized nature of the need to move the body and the occurrence in association with use of dopamine-receptor antagonists.
- *Painful legs and moving toes* have neither a clear circadian pattern nor the sense of an urge to move.
- *PLMD* represents a disorder present only in sleep without any of the essential diagnostic features of RLS.
- *Sleep related leg cramps* are worse at night, relieved by movement, and, in rare cases, interpreted as an urge to move; these leg cramps always involve a muscle hardening or pain and usually require strong stretching of the muscle more than moving of the leg to relieve symptoms.
- *Pain* involving the legs occurs with several conditions, including arthritis, vascular problems,

sports injuries, and neuropathy. These pains can have a nocturnal presentation and may be worse at rest, but improvement with movement usually entails more exercise than simple movement of the leg. The urge to move, if present at all, usually stems from awareness that movement produces relief rather than the strong primary urgency of movement felt with RLS. The presence of pain, however, does not exclude a diagnosis of RLS, since many patients with RLS report their RLS symptoms as pain.

Diagnostic Criteria for

Periodic Limb Movement Disorder 327.51

A. Polysomnography demonstrates repetitive, highly stereotyped, limb movements that are:

    i. 0.5 to 5 seconds in duration

    ii. Of amplitude greater than or equal to 25% of toe dorsiflexion during calibration

    iii. In a sequence of four or more movements

    iv. Separated by an interval of more than five seconds (from limb-movement onset to limb-movement onset) and less than 90 seconds (typically there is an interval of 20 to 40 seconds)

B. The PLMS Index exceeds five per hour in children and 15 per hour in most adult cases

Note: The PLMS Index must be interpreted in the context of a patient's sleep related complaint. In adults, normative values higher than the previously accepted value of five per hour have been found in studies that did not exclude RERAs (using sensitive respiratory monitoring) and other causes for PLMS. New data suggest a partial overlap of PLMS Index values between symptomatic and asymptomatic individuals, emphasizing the importance of clinical context over an absolute cutoff value.

C. There is clinical sleep disturbance or a complaint of daytime fatigue.

Note: If PLMS are present without clinical sleep disturbance, the PLMS can be noted as a polysomnographic finding, but criteria are not met for a diagnosis of PLMD.

D. The PLMs are not better explained by another current sleep disorder, medical or neurological disorder, mental disorder, medication use, or substance use disorder (e.g., PLMs at the termination of cyclically occurring apneas should not be counted as true PLMS or PLMD).

Alternate Names

Nocturnal myoclonus, periodic leg movements in sleep.

Essential Features

PLMD is characterized by periodic episodes of repetitive, highly stereotyped PLMS and by clinical sleep disturbance that cannot be accounted for by another primary sleep disorder. PLMS occur most frequently in the lower extremities. They typically involve extension of the big toe, often in combination with partial flexion of the ankle, the knee, and sometimes the hip. Similar movements can occur in the upper limbs. Individual movements may be associated with an autonomic arousal, a cortical arousal, or an awakening. Typically, the patient is unaware of the limb movements or the sleep disruption. An arousal may precede, coincide with, or follow the limb movement. Marked night-to-night variability in the number of movements has been documented. In some cases, the periodic limb movements may also occur while awake and are designated PLMW. A clinical history of sleep onset or sleep maintenance problems, or both, is most consistently reported in association with PLMD. Many individuals with PLMD report having unrefreshing sleep, and some have a subjective complaint of excessive daytime sleepiness. Clinical symptoms, bed-partner observations, or parental reports for children may help in the clinical indication of PLMD. It is necessary to integrate a detailed clinical history and the polysomnographic findings to assess the role of this phenomenon as a sleep disorder. A sensitive technique, such as pressure transducer airflow monitoring, should be used to monitor breathing during polysomnography to reasonably exclude sleep related breathing disorders as the direct cause of the PLMS. When independent PLMS are present in patients with SRBDs, a separate diagnosis of PLMD may be considered if the PLMS persist despite adequate continuous positive airway pressure and a clinical sleep disturbance remains that is not otherwise explained. When PLMS and a specific insomnia syndrome are present, then a clinical decision regarding the role of PLMS in the generation or exacerbation of insomnia symptoms must be made.

Associated Features

A sustained clinical response to dopaminergic therapy is supportive of the diagnosis of PLMD.

Predisposing & Precipitating Factors

PLMS are commonly found in association with three well-defined primary sleep disorders: RLS, RBD, and narcolepsy. Research studies indicate that five or more PLMS occur per hour in 80% to 90% of patients with RLS, in about 70% with RBD, and in 45% to 65% with narcolepsy. PLMS are so common in RLS that they are considered to be supportive of an RLS diagnosis when other RLS symptoms are present.

Polysomnographic & Other Objective Findings

PLMS typically occur in discrete episodes that last from a few minutes to an hour. Movements of the upper limbs may be sampled if clinically indicated. The movements may affect one or, more typically, both of the lower limbs but not necessarily in a symmetric or simultaneous pattern. Simultaneous movements in both legs are counted as one movement. Contractions occurring during wakefulness, before the onset of stage 1 sleep, are not counted as part of the sleep disorder but can be scored separately as PLMW. Periodic limb movements may be associated with EEG (cortical) arousals or with awakenings. The movements should be reported as an index of total sleep time called the PLMS Index. The PLMS Index is the number of periodic limb movements per hour of total sleep time, as determined by polysomnography. The PLMS Index should exceed norms for age to be considered pathologic. The PLMS Arousal Index is the number of PLMs associated with a cortical arousal, expressed per hour of total sleep time.

Differential Diagnosis

- *Sleep starts (hypnic jerks)* need to be differentiated from PLMD. Sleep starts typically are limited to the transition from wakefulness to sleep, are not periodic, and are briefer (20 to 100 milliseconds) than PLMS.
- *Normal phasic REM activity* is limited to REM sleep, typically occurs in 5- to 15-second clusters, and is usually associated with bursts of REMs.
- *Fragmentary myoclonus* is characterized by EMG activity that is briefer (75 to 150 milliseconds), more variable in duration, and less periodic than PLMS. Fragmentary myoclonus is primarily an EMG diagnosis with little or no visible movement.
- PLMD must be differentiated from movements associated with *nocturnal epileptic seizures*

and *myoclonic epilepsy* and from a number of forms of *myoclonus* seen while awake, such as in *Alzheimer's disease, Creutzfeldt-Jakob disease,* and *other neuropathologic conditions*. However, in these disorders, the involuntary movements are prominent during the daytime, often do not disappear with activity, are prominent in the arms and other body parts in addition to the legs, and do not display the periodicity seen with PLMD.

Diagnostic Criteria for

Sleep Related Leg Cramps 327.52

A. A painful sensation in the leg or foot is associated with sudden muscle hardness or tightness indicating a strong muscle contraction.

B. The painful muscle contractions in the legs or feet occur during the sleep period, although they may arise from either wakefulness or sleep.

C. The pain is relieved by forceful stretching of the affected muscles, releasing the contraction.

D. The disorder is not better explained by another current sleep disorder, medical or neurological disorder, medication use, or substance use disorder.

Alternate Names
Leg cramps, "charley horse."

Essential Features
Sleep related leg cramps are painful sensations caused by sudden and intense involuntary contractions of muscles or muscle groups, usually in the calf or small muscles of the foot, occurring during the sleep period. They may arise from either wakefulness or sleep. Sleep related leg cramps usually start abruptly but may in some cases be preceded by a less painful warning sensation. The muscle contractions last for a few seconds up to several minutes and then remit spontaneously; the frequency of sleep related leg cramps varies considerably from less than yearly to multiple episodes every night. The cramp can be relieved by strongly stretching the affected muscle and sometimes also by local massage, application of heat, or movement of the affected limb.

Associated Features
Tenderness and discomfort in the muscle may persist for several hours after the cramping. The muscle cramp not only causes pain, but also reduces sleep.

Demographics
Sleep related leg cramps appear to occur at any age but are more common and frequent in the elderly.

Differential Diagnosis
- *Chronic myelopathy, peripheral neuropathy, akathisia, muscular pain-fasciculation syndromes*, and *disorders of calcium metabolism* should be differentiated by clinical history and physical examination.
- Sleep related leg cramps may coexist with other sleep disorders, such as *PLMD* or *SRBDs*.
- *RLS* is sometimes confused with sleep related leg cramps because both present with leg pains during the sleep period. RLS involves an urge to move not commonly seen with sleep related leg cramps. RLS usually does not involve a sensation of pain, but, when reported, the pain from RLS is at least partly relieved almost immediately by any significant movement of the leg. In contrast, relieving the pain from leg cramps requires both more time and more vigorous stretching of the muscle.

Diagnostic Criteria for

Sleep Related Bruxism 327.53

A. The patient reports or is aware of tooth-grinding sounds or tooth clenching during sleep.

B. One or more of the following is present:
   - i. Abnormal wear of the teeth
   - ii. Jaw muscle discomfort, fatigue, or pain and jaw lock upon awakening
   - iii. Masseter muscle hypertrophy upon voluntary forceful clenching

C. The disorder is not better explained by another current sleep disorder, medical or neurological disorder, medication use, or substance use disorder.

Alternate Names
Nocturnal tooth grinding.

Essential Features

Sleep related bruxism is characterized by grinding or clenching of the teeth during sleep, usually associated with sleep arousals. In sleep, jaw contraction frequently occurs. This contraction can take two forms: isolated sustained jaw clenching, termed *tonic contractions*, or a series of repetitive (phasic) muscle contractions termed *rhythmic masticatory muscle activity*. When these contractions are particularly strong during sleep, they frequently produce tooth-grinding sounds and are referred to as *sleep related bruxism*. This condition can lead to abnormal wear of the teeth, tooth pain, jaw muscle pain, or temporal headache. Severe sleep related bruxism may also result in sleep disruption. The disorder is typically brought to dental or medical attention because of the tooth damage or disturbing sounds. Less commonly, it may present as a cause of disturbed sleep. Temporomandibular joint pain, accompanied by limited jaw movement, is not a rare consequence. Sleep related bruxism without clear cause is termed primary, whereas secondary sleep related bruxism may be associated with the use of psychoactive medications, recreational drugs or a variety of medical disorders. Treatment-induced secondary sleep related bruxism is termed iatrogenic.

Associated Features

Additional symptoms include a variety of unpleasant muscle and tooth sensations, limitation of jaw movements, oral and facial pain, and headache. Tooth wear, fractured teeth, and buccal lacerations may occur.

Polysomnographic & Other Objective Findings

To test for sleep related bruxism, there must be a minimum of one masseter muscle monitor with audio recording to associate muscular activity with grinding sound production. In routine clinical polysomnography, bruxism is suggested by either a phasic pattern of masseter and temporalis muscle activity at 1 Hz frequency lasting 0.25 to 2 seconds, sustained tonic activity lasting longer than two seconds, or a mixed pattern. An episode begins after at least a three-second interval with no muscle activity. Video monitoring can show the bruxing movements. A diagnosis of sleep related bruxism is given in the presence of at least four episodes per hour of sleep or 25 individual muscle bursts per hour of sleep and a minimum of two audible tooth-grinding episodes per sleep-recording session in the absence of associated abnormal EEG activity (e.g., epilepsy).

Differential Diagnosis

- The disorder seldom poses diagnostic problems, but evaluation for temporomandibular disorders or dental structures is indicated. The other facio-mandibular activities to differentiate from sleep related bruxism are *facio-mandibular myoclonus* (observed in approximately 10% of frequent tooth grinders), *respiratory disturbances, RBD, abnormal swallowing, sleep terrors, confusional arousals, daytime dyskinetic movements* persisting in sleep involving the jaw (dystonia, tremor, chorea, dyskinesia), and *sleep related epilepsy* (rare). The rhythmic jaw movements associated with partial complex or generalized seizure disorders need to be considered in the differential diagnosis, although a presentation of epilepsy as relatively isolated sleep related bruxism is very rare.

Sleep Related Rhythmic Movement Disorder

Please see the Pediatric section of the Manual for this diagnosis.

ICSD-2 Section VII, "Isolated Symptoms, Apparently Normal Variants and Unresolved Issues," is not included in this handbook.

VIII. Other Sleep Disorders

Other Physiological (Organic) Sleep Disorder 327.80

A sleep disorder is temporarily classified here if it cannot be placed elsewhere in the *ICSD-2* and the expectation is that a final diagnosis will have a physiological or medical basis. This diagnosis is also used as a permanent classification for sleep disorders that cannot be placed anywhere else in the *ICSD-2*, but are believed to be due to physiological or medical factors. This is also the default category in which to place sleep disorders not classifiable elsewhere, when there is no evidence whether the sleep disorder has a medical, a substance, or a psychiatric etiology.

Other Sleep Disorder Not Due to Substance or Known Physiological Condition 307.40

A sleep disorder is classified here if it cannot be placed anywhere else in the *ICSD-2* and a suggestion exists that it is based on psychiatric or behavioral factors.

Diagnostic Criteria for

Environmental Sleep Disorder 307.48

A. The patient complains of insomnia, daytime fatigue, or a parasomnia. In cases in which daytime fatigue is present, the daytime fatigue may occur as a result of the accompanying insomnia or as a result of poor quality of nocturnal sleep.

B. The complaint is temporally associated with the introduction of a physically measurable stimulus or environmental circumstance that disturbs sleep.

C. It is the physical properties, rather than the psychological meaning of the environmental factor, that accounts for the sleep complaint.

D. The sleep disturbance is not better explained by another sleep disorder, medical or neurological disorder, mental disorder, medication use, or substance use disorder.

Alternate Names

Environment-induced somnolence, environmental insomnia, environment-induced sleep disorder, noise-induced sleep disturbance, temperature-induced sleep disturbance, bed partner-related sleep disorder, hospital-induced sleep disorder, sleep disorder associated with forced vigilance.

Essential Features

Environmental sleep disorder is a sleep disturbance due to a disturbing environmental factor that causes a complaint of either insomnia or daytime fatigue and somnolence.

Associated Features

Secondary symptoms may result, including deficits in concentration, attention, and cognitive performance; reduced vigilance; daytime fatigue; malaise; depressed mood; and irritability. Also, certain environmental factors have been shown to reduce slow-wave sleep, which may result in muscle aches, social withdrawal, and somatic preoccupation.

Differential Diagnosis

- Environmental sleep disorder must be differentiated from *inadequate sleep hygiene; behaviorally induced insufficient sleep syndrome; psychophysiological insomnia; insomnia not due to substance or known physiological condition, unspecified; circadian rhythm sleep disorder, irregular sleep-wake type; OSA; CSA; narcolepsy; idiopathic hypersomnia; circadian rhythm sleep disorder, delayed sleep phase type; adjustment insomnia; and behavioral insomnia of childhood, sleep-onset association type.*
- Of all these disorders, the insomnia of environmental sleep disorder is most closely aligned with the *behavioral insomnia of childhood, sleep-onset association type.* When the sleep environment is noxious, the correct diagnosis is environmental sleep disorder. When insomnia occurs in children only because the sleep setting is unfamiliar, the diagnosis of *behavioral insomnia of childhood, sleep-onset association type*, should be entertained.

PEDIATRIC SECTION

Diagnostic Criteria for

Behavioral Insomnia of Childhood (Sleep-Onset Type) v69.5

A. A child's symptoms meet the criteria for insomnia based upon reports of parents or other adult caregivers.

B. The child shows a pattern consistent with sleep-onset association with the following symptoms:

    i. Falling asleep is an extended process that requires special conditions

    ii. Sleep-onset associations are highly problematic or demanding

    iii. In the absence of the associated conditions, sleep onset is significantly delayed or sleep is otherwise disrupted

    iv. Awakenings require caregiver intervention for the child to return to sleep

C. The sleep disturbance is not better explained by another sleep disorder, medical or neurological disorder, mental disorder, medication use, or substance use disorder.

Diagnostic Criteria for

Behavioral Insomnia of Childhood (Limit-Setting Type) v69.5

A. A child's symptoms meet the criteria for insomnia based upon reports of parents or other adult caregivers.

B. The child shows a pattern consistent with limit-setting type with the following symptoms:

    i. The individual has difficulty initiating or maintaining sleep

    ii. The individual stalls or refuses to go to bed at an appropriate time or refuses to return to bed following a nighttime awakening

    iii. The caregiver demonstrates insufficient or inappropriate limit setting to establish appropriate sleeping behavior in the child

C. The sleep disturbance is not better explained by another sleep disorder, medical or neurological disorder, mental disorder, medication use, or substance use disorder.

Alternate Names

Childhood insomnia, limit-setting sleep disorder, sleep-onset association disorder.

Essential Features

Sleep difficulties are the result of inappropriate sleep associations or inadequate limit setting. *Sleep-onset Association Type.* This type of behavioral insomnia is characterized by reliance on inappropriate sleep associations and usually presents as frequent nighttime awakenings. In this disorder, the process of falling asleep is associated with a specific form of stimulation (e.g., rocking, watching television), object (e.g., bottle), or setting (e.g., lighted room, parents' bed). The child is unable to fall asleep within a reasonable time in the absence of these conditions. *Limit-setting Type.* Stalling or refusing to go to sleep characterizes limit-setting sleep disorder. If and when a caregiver enforces limits, sleep comes quickly; otherwise, sleep onset is delayed. The bedtime problems often result from parental difficulties in setting limits and managing behavior.

Associated Features

The sleep disturbance may be accompanied by daytime behavioral problems, limit-setting difficulties during the day, or both. In addition, the nighttime sleep disturbance often results in poor parental sleep and associated daytime impairment.

Differential Diagnosis

- A *circadian rhythm sleep disorder, delayed sleep phase type*, or an inappropriately early bedtime will usually present as a bedtime problem. Conditions such as *circadian rhythm sleep disorder, irregular sleep-wake type* and *inadequate sleep hygiene* may present with multiple awakenings as well, but, in these cases, rapid parental intervention does not ensure rapid return to sleep.
- *Anxiety disorders* can present as bedtime difficulties; however, a child with an anxiety disorder at night typically exhibits anxiety symptoms at other times of the day. Medication effects may also lead to delayed sleep onset.
- An underlying *medical disorder* including gastroesophageal reflux, asthma, milk intolerance, and pain (such as otitis) can also account for difficulties falling asleep and staying asleep.
- Other sleep disorders such as *OSA*, *RLS*, and *PLMD* should also be considered. If the disorder has been present for less than 3 months, the differentiation must be made from *adjustment insomnia*.

Diagnostic Criteria for

Primary Sleep Apnea of Infancy (formerly Primary Sleep Apnea of Newborn) 770.81

A. *Apnea of Prematurity.* Prolonged central respiratory pauses of 20 seconds or more in duration (or shorter-duration events that include obstructive or mixed respiratory patterns and are associated with a significant physiologic compromise, including decrease in heart rate, hypoxemia, clinical symptoms, or need for nursing intervention), are recorded in an infant younger than 37 weeks conceptional age.

B. *Apnea of Infancy.* Prolonged central respiratory pauses of 20 seconds or more in duration (or shorter-duration events that include obstructive or mixed respiratory patterns and are associated with bradycardia, cyanosis, pallor, or marked hypotonia), are recorded in an infant with a conceptional age of 37 weeks or older.

C. *For either diagnosis,* the disorder is not better explained by another current sleep disorder, medical or neurological disorder, or medication.

Alternate Names

Apnea of prematurity.

Essential Features

Primary sleep apnea of infancy is characterized by prolonged central, mixed, or obstructive apneas or hypopneas associated with physiological compromise (hypoxemia, bradycardia, or the need for intervention such as stimulation or resuscitation). It is a disorder of respiratory control that can be either a developmental problem associated with immaturity of the brainstem respiratory centers or secondary to other medical conditions (e.g., anemia, infection, hypoxemia, metabolic disturbances, gastroesophageal reflux, drugs, or anesthesia) that produce apnea by direct depression of central respiratory control, disturbance of oxygen delivery, or ventilation defects.

Associated Features

Primary sleep apnea of infancy is state dependent and the frequency of respiratory events increases during active (REM) sleep. Note that a small upper airway will exaggerate the obstructive elements of this disorder.

Familial Patterns

Familial patterns of primary sleep apnea of infancy have not been demonstrated.

Onset, Course, & Complications

In preterm infants, primary sleep apnea of infancy is rare on day one of life, and its presence usually signals another illness. More typical onset occurs between the second and seventh days. Primary sleep apnea of infancy in the preterm infant usually ceases by 37 weeks conceptional age but may persist for several weeks beyond term, especially in infants born before 28 weeks post-conception.

Polysomnographic & Other Objective Findings

Mixed sleep apnea is the most frequently observed type of apnea in small premature infants, accounting for 50% to 75% of all apneas in premature infants; obstructive-type events account for 10% to 20% of events; and pure central events, 10% to 25%. On the other hand, apnea in larger premature and term infants weighing more than 2000g at birth is predominantly central, unless there is an underlying upper-airway problem leading to a more obstructive presentation. Polysomnography is the gold standard for the diagnosis of unexplained problematic sleep disordered breathing in infants, although limited-channel studies may be quite useful for specific clinical scenarios. Decisions about diagnostic testing strategies depend on the pertinent clinical questions and clinical correlates for the individual patient. However, full polysomnography with a complete seizure montage, esophageal pH sensor, or both may be diagnostically appropriate for problem cases with persistent symptoms.

Differential Diagnosis

- Primary sleep apnea of infancy should be distinguished from *periodic breathing*, which has a pattern of regular cycles of regular respiration for 10 to 18 seconds in length, interrupted by pauses that are three seconds or longer in duration.
- Primary sleep apnea of infancy should also be distinguished from the *normal respiratory pauses* that occur during sleep. Normative respiratory data from several large studies show that healthy asymptomatic infants have all types of self-limited apneas, mainly during active sleep. Short central respiratory pauses are commonly seen in infants, either as isolated events or

after sigh breaths or movements.

- Primary sleep apnea of infancy should be distinguished from the popular clinical term, *ALTE*, which is not a specific diagnosis but an ill-defined constellation of parent-reported apnea symptoms that range in severity from benign to life threatening. Infants with ALTE-type symptoms are a heterogeneous group. In 40% to 50% of all cases, a careful focused clinical assessment, including history, physical examination, judicious laboratory evaluation, and occasionally a period of inpatient observation, will identify a specific diagnosis such as a respiratory infection, gastroesophageal reflux, seizure, breath-holding spell, or even normal respiratory behavior misinterpreted as abnormal.

- *Sleep apnea* in a preterm infant or term infant who is less than 44 weeks postconceptional age is usually related to immaturity or developmental delay in respiratory control and almost always resolves with maturation beyond that age. When sleep apnea occurs after that time, especially when repeated physiological compromise (significant gas exchange abnormalities, impaired consciousness, cardiorespiratory arrest, or cardiovascular collapse) is reported, a diagnosis must be aggressively pursued.

- Recurrent severe infant sleep apnea is usually due to other comorbid conditions, including a *small upper airway, gastroesophageal reflux, metabolic disease*, or unrecognized neurological conditions such as *seizures, brainstem malformation, or neurodegenerative condition*.

- Another diagnostic consideration is a form of child abuse (*Munchausen's syndrome by proxy*) manifest as imposed upper airway obstruction or attempted suffocation.

- Primary sleep apnea of infancy should be disassociated from the postmortem diagnosis of sudden infant death syndrome. *SIDS* is defined as "the sudden death of an infant less than one year of age that remains unexplained after a thorough case investigation, including performance of a complete autopsy, examination of the death scene, and review of the clinical history." Although a small percentage of SIDS victims experience apnea symptoms prior to death, primary apnea in the newborn or infant has not been established as an independent risk factor for SIDS.

Diagnostic Criteria for

Obstructive Sleep Apnea, Pediatric 327.23

A. The caregiver reports snoring, labored or obstructed breathing, or both snoring and labored or obstructed breathing during the child's sleep.

B. The caregiver of the child reports observing at least one of the following:

    i. Paradoxical inward rib-cage motion during inspiration

    ii. Movement arousals

    iii. Diaphoresis

    iv. Neck hyperextension during sleep

    v. Excessive daytime sleepiness, hyperactivity, or aggressive behavior

    vi. A slow rate of growth

    vii. Morning headaches

    viii. Secondary enuresis

C. Polysomnographic recording demonstrates one or more scoreable respiratory event per hour (i.e., apnea or hypopnea of at least two respiratory cycles in duration)

Note: *Very few normative data are available for hypopneas, and the data that are available have been obtained using a variety of methodologies. These criteria may be modified in the future once more comprehensive data become available.*

D. Polysomnographic recording demonstrates either i or ii.

    i. At least one of the following is observed:

        a. Frequent arousals from sleep associated with increased respiratory effort

        b. Arterial oxygen desaturation in association with the apneic episodes

        c. Hypercapnia during sleep

        d. Markedly negative esophageal pressure swings

    ii. Periods of hypercapnia, desaturation, or hypercapnia and desaturation during sleep associated with snoring, paradoxical inward rib-cage motion during inspiration, and at least one of the following:

        a. Frequent arousals from sleep

        b. Markedly negative esophageal pressure swings

E. The disorder is not better explained by another current sleep disorder, medical or neurological disorder, medication use, or substance use disorder.

Essential Features

Pediatric OSA is characterized by prolonged partial upper airway obstruction, intermittent complete or partial obstruction (obstructive apnea or hypopnea), or both prolonged and intermittent obstruction that disrupts normal ventilation during sleep, normal sleep patterns, or both. Children with OSA may demonstrate several breathing patterns during sleep. Some children have cyclic episodes of obstructive apnea, similar to that of adults with the syndrome. However, some patients, particularly younger children, have a pattern of obstructive hypoventilation, which consists of long periods of persistent partial upper airway obstruction associated with hypercarbia, arterial oxygen desaturation, or hypercarbia and desaturation. Some children may manifest a pattern of UARS similar to that seen in adults, including snoring without identifiable airflow obstruction and increasingly negative esophageal pressure swings and arousals. Most children with OSA present with a history of snoring and difficulty breathing during sleep. Snoring is usually loud and may be punctuated by pauses and gasps, with associated movements or arousal from sleep. However, some patients, particularly infants and those who are weak, may not snore. Patients with obstructive hypoventilation often have continuous snoring without pauses or arousals.

Associated Features

Hypoxemia and hypercapnia are often present during sleep and may be severe. A prominent sinus arrhythmia is often present, although other arrhythmias are rare. Secondary enuresis may occur. Breathing during wakefulness is normal, although mouth breathing secondary to adenoidal hypertrophy may be present. Excessive daytime sleepiness may be present, especially in older children and adolescents, but is seen less commonly in children than in adults with OSA.

Demographics

The prevalence of OSA is approximately 2% in otherwise-normal young children

Predisposing & Precipitating Factors

Children with OSA generally have larger tonsils and adenoids than do other children; obesity also appears to be a risk factor in children. Children with craniofacial abnormalities, specifically micrognathia, midfacial hypoplasia, and associated hypotonia, are at risk. Children with neuromuscular diseases often have upper airway muscle weakness, which predisposes the airway to collapse. Children with cerebral palsy may be predisposed to OSA because of spasticity of the upper airway muscles. Infants with gastroesophageal reflux may develop upper airway edema, resulting in obstructive events.

Familial Patterns

There is strong evidence for an increased risk of OSA in children with other affected family members.

Polysomnographic & Other Objective Findings

In children, obstructive apneas lasting two respiratory cycles or longer are scored. EEG arousals may or may not be present following apneas. Sleep architecture is usually normal. Apneas and partial obstructions occur primarily during REM sleep, and breathing may be totally normal during NREM sleep. Esophageal pressure measurements, when obtained, are often markedly negative.

Differential Diagnosis

- Pediatric OSA must be differentiated from primary *snoring.* This distinction cannot usually be made clinically but is based on polysomnography. Children with primary snoring do not have apneas, gas-exchange abnormalities, or frequent arousals on polysomnography.
- *CSA* can be differentiated from OSA by the lack of chest or abdominal wall movement associated with the central apneas. Mixed apneas may be seen and are included in the diagnosis of OSA.
- Children with *fixed upper airway obstruction* due to structural abnormalities will obstruct while both awake and asleep and will have stridor rather than snoring.
- *OSA* in children must be distinguished from *nonobstructive alveolar hypoventilation.* Children with lung or chest wall disease may have desaturation and hypercapnia during sleep. It may be difficult to separate nonobstructive hypoventilation and desaturation from OSA, especially because the two conditions may coexist. In general, children with nonobstructive hypoventilation will not snore and will not have paradoxical inward rib-cage motion during inspiration, although the latter may be present in children with neuromuscular disease.
- OSA must be differentiated from other causes of sleepiness such as *narcolepsy, insufficient sleep,* and *PLMD.*
- *Sleep related epilepsy* may mimic obstructive apnea during sleep and may be indistinguishable from OSA without the appropriate EEG monitoring, especially in infants who may have only subtle motor components of seizures.

Diagnostic Criteria for

Congenital Central Alveolar Hypoventilation Syndrome 327.25

A. The patient exhibits shallow breathing, or cyanosis and apnea, of perinatal onset during sleep.

Note: *In severely affected infants, consequences of hypoxia, including pulmonary hypertension and cor pulmonale, may also be present.*

B. Hypoventilation is worse during sleep than during wakefulness.

C. The rebreathing ventilatory response to hypoxia and hypercapnia is absent or diminished.

D. Polysomnographic monitoring during sleep demonstrates severe hypercapnia and hypoxia, predominantly without apnea.

E. The disorder is not better explained by another current sleep disorder, medical or neurological disorder, medication use, or substance use disorder.

Alternate Names

The term, "Ondine's curse" is not recommended due to its negative connotations.

Essential Features

Congenital central alveolar hypoventilation syndrome (CCHS) is the failure of automatic central control of breathing. CCHS is characterized by the onset of hypoventilation, usually in infancy. The hypoventilation is worse during sleep than wakefulness and is unexplained by primary pulmonary, neurological, or metabolic disease. CCHS presents in an otherwise normal-appearing infant who does not breathe spontaneously or breathes only shallowly or erratically. In most infants, a problem is evident at birth. The infant requires intubation and then cannot be weaned from mechanically assisted ventilation, despite appearing vigorous and having a normal chest radiogram. Some infants may appear to breathe adequately on clinical examination but experience episodes of hypoventilation (not necessarily apnea) characterized by hypoxemia and hypercapnia. These patients may occasionally present later in life with cyanosis, an apparent life-threatening event, cor pulmonale, or hypoxic neurological damage. Most patients with CCHS have severe hypoventilation during sleep, to the point that they require mechanically assisted ventilation, although this state-dependent difference may not be apparent during early infancy. Some patients hypoventilate during wakefulness as well as during sleep and require continuous ventilatory support. Most patients with CCHS do not require ventilatory support during wakefulness but may have subtle abnormalities in gas exchange when physically inactive.

Associated Features
Associated abnormalities include Hirschsprung's disease in approximately 16% of patients with CCHS, autonomic dysfunction (e.g., decreased heart-rate variability or hypotension), neural tumors (e.g., ganglioneuromas or ganglioneuroblastomas), swallowing dysfunction during early years, and ocular abnormalities (e.g., strabismus). Most patients are cognitively normal, although developmental delay may be present, especially in patients in whom the hypoventilation has not been well controlled.

Familial Patterns
Recently, it has been established that the vast majority of cases of CCHS are due to de novo mutations in the *PHOX2B* gene. This appears to be transmitted as a dominant trait with incomplete penetrance.

Polysomnographic & Other Objective Findings
Gas-exchange abnormalities may progress as the sleep period lengthens. In contrast to findings in most types of sleep related breathing disorders, abnormalities may be more severe during slow-wave sleep than during REM sleep. Patients may not arouse from sleep despite severe gas-exchange abnormalities. CSA may be present but is not usually noted. Paradoxical breathing and snoring do not typically occur. Patients with CCHS have blunted rebreathing hypoxic and hypercapnic responses, although they may respond to transient ventilatory challenges of the peripheral chemoreceptors. Arterial blood gases may be normal during wakefulness but will be abnormal if obtained from an arterial line during sleep. In patients with chronically untreated or poorly controlled CCHS, a compensated respiratory acidosis may be present. In these patients, polycythemia may be present, and the serum bicarbonate level may be elevated. Computed tomography and magnetic resonance imaging scans of the head are normal.

Clinical & Pathophysiological Subtypes

CCHS is a heterogeneous disease. Affected individuals include patients who hypoventilate severely during both wakefulness and sleep, those who hypoventilate severely only during sleep, patients with and without Hirschsprung's disease, and patients with and without neural tumors. A group of patients with late-onset central hypoventilation associated with hypothalamic abnormalities has also been described. These patients typically present at two to four years of age with hypoventilation, onset of morbid obesity, and other hypothalamic abnormalities, such as endocrine abnormalities

Differential Diagnosis

- CCHS must be distinguished from other forms of *central hypoventilation*, such as central hypoventilation due to Arnold-Chiari malformation, other causes of central nervous system disturbance such as trauma or tumors, metabolic conditions such as Leigh disease, or obesity hypoventilation syndrome.
- CCHS must also be distinguished from *hypoventilation secondary to muscle weakness* due to conditions such as diaphragmatic paralysis or muscular dystrophy.
- The diagnosis of CCHS is usually one of exclusion after physical examination and laboratory tests exclude other causes of hypoventilation. Infants presenting with apnea or an ALTE due to causes such as gastroesophageal reflux may be thought to have CCHS. However, these infants typically have intermittent episodes of apnea rather than sustained hypoventilation, and the episodes typically resolve once the primary cause has been treated. Patients presenting with cor pulmonale may be misdiagnosed as having congenital heart disease.

Diagnostic Criteria for

Sleep Enuresis 788.36

Primary
A. The patient is older than five years of age.
B. The patient exhibits recurrent involuntary voiding during sleep, occurring at least twice a week.
C. The patient has never been consistently dry during sleep.

Secondary
A. The patient is older than five years of age.
B. The patient exhibits recurrent involuntary voiding during sleep, occurring at least twice a week.
C. The patient has previously been consistently dry during sleep for at least six months.

Alternate Names
Enuresis nocturna; nocturnal bedwetting.

Essential Features
Sleep enuresis is characterized by recurrent involuntary voiding that occurs during sleep.

Associated Features
Involuntary voiding during wakefulness may be associated with sleep enuresis and, if present, generally points toward an organic etiology. Sleep enuresis can occur in association with diabetes and urinary tract infection. It may occur in individuals with nocturnal epilepsy. Among older adults, sleep enuresis may be associated with symptoms of congestive heart failure, OSA, depression, and dementia.

Familial Patterns
There is often a high prevalence of enuresis among the parents, siblings, and other relatives of the child with primary enuresis. The reported prevalence is 77% when both parents were enuretic as children and 44% when one parent has a history of enuresis.

Polysomnographic & Other Objective Findings
In primary and secondary sleep enuresis, enuretic episodes can occur in all sleep stages, during nocturnal wakefulness, and in association with transient arousals. Laboratory and urologic studies should be pursued only if there is a clear history suggestive of a specific problem. Routine laboratory tests generally include only a urinalysis and urine culture. Polysomnographic monitoring is

only indicated in the evaluation of secondary sleep enuresis when one suspects another sleep disorder such as OSA or sleep related epilepsy as the cause of the enuresis.

Differential Diagnosis

- Primary sleep enuresis is diagnosed by exclusion when secondary sleep enuresis has been ruled out. Individuals with suspected primary sleep enuresis should have a physical examination that includes a urinalysis, complete enuresis history, and a sleep history.
- Causes of secondary enuresis can be organic, medical, or psychologic. Organic pathology of the urinary tract is more likely if the child has daytime enuresis, abnormalities in the initiation of micturition, or abnormal urinary flow. *Urinary tract infection, diabetes mellitus, diabetes insipidus, epilepsy, sickle cell disease,* and *neurologic disorders* can all cause enuresis.

Diagnostic Criteria for

Restless Legs Syndrome 333.99

Diagnosis in Pediatric Patients (Age 2 to 12 Years)
A alone *or* B and C satisfy the criteria:

A. The child meets all four essential adult criteria for RLS listed previously and relates a description, in his or her own words, that is consistent with leg discomfort.

B. The child meets all four essential adult criteria for RLS listed previously but does not relate a description in his or her own words that is consistent with leg discomfort.

C. The child has at least two of the following three findings:
  i. A sleep disturbance for age
  ii. A biological parent or sibling with definite RLS
  iii. A polysomnographically documented periodic limb movement index of five or more movements per hour of sleep

Note: Criteria for probable and possible childhood RLS have been developed for research purposes and are included in a National Institutes of Health diagnostic workshop report.

Please see adult Restless Legs Syndrome section in Chapter VI for further details.

Sleep Related Rhythmic Movement Disorder 327.59

A. The patient exhibits repetitive, stereotyped, and rhythmic motor behaviors.

B. The movements involve large muscle groups.

C. The movements are predominantly sleep related, occurring near nap or bedtime, or when the individual appears drowsy or asleep.

D. The behaviors result in a significant complaint as manifest by at least one of the following:

      i. Interference with normal sleep

      ii. Significant impairment in daytime function

      iii. Self-inflicted bodily injury that requires medical treatment (or would result in injury if preventable measures were not used)

E. The rhythmic movements are not better explained by another current sleep disorder, medical or neurological disorder, mental disorder, medication use, or substance use disorder.

Alternate Names

Body rocking, head banging, *jactatio capitis nocturna*.

Essential Features

Sleep related rhythmic movement disorder (RMD) is characterized by repetitive, stereotyped, and rhythmic motor behaviors (not tremors) that occur predominantly during drowsiness or sleep and involve large muscle groups. The occurrence of significant clinical consequences differentiates RMD from developmentally normal sleep related movements. Typically seen in infants and children, RMD comprises several subtypes. *Body rocking* may involve the entire body, with the child on hands and knees, or it may be limited to the torso, with the child sitting. *Head banging* often occurs with the child prone, repeatedly lifting the head or entire upper torso, and forcibly banging the head back down into the pillow or mattress. Alternately, the child may sit with the back of the head against the headboard or wall, repeatedly banging the occiput. Combining head banging and body rocking, the child may rock on hands and knees, banging the vertex or frontal region of the head into the headboard or wall. *Head rolling* consists of side-to-side head movements, usually with the child in the supine position. Less common rhythmic movement forms include body rolling, leg banging, or leg rolling. Rhythmic humming or inarticulate sounds often accompany the body, head, or limb movements and may be quite loud. Episodes often occur near sleep onset, although they may also occur at any time during the night and even during quiet wakeful activities. The movement frequency can vary, but the rate is usually between 0.5 per second and 2 per second. Duration of the individual movement clusters also varies but generally is less than 15 minutes. Children who have sufficient language development to be asked about event recall in the morning are typically amnesic for the episodes. Sleep related rhythmic movements are common in normal infants and children. Without evidence for significant consequences, the movements alone should not be considered a disorder.

Differential Diagnosis

- *RMD* must be distinguished from other repetitive movements involving restricted small muscle groups, such as *sleep related bruxism*, *thumb sucking*, and *rhythmic sucking of a pacifier or the lips*, as well as other specifically-defined rhythmic movements of sleep, such as *hypnagogic foot tremor*.
- Children with *autism* and *pervasive developmental disorders* often exhibit repetitive behaviors, but these movements typically occur during wakefulness.

INDEX TERMS

L

M

N

O

P